NHIA ACT
Advanced Certificate Training

AF770349

Advanced Certificate Training

Sterile Compounding

Abby Roth, BS, CMQ/OE

A National Home Infusion Association Publication

The National Home Infusion Association (NHIA) produces educational resources to aid good clinical practice that reflects the input of its members and experienced clinicians in the field. The information offered in NHIA resources is intended as a guide for information purposes only and does not replace or remove clinical judgment or the professional care and duty necessary for each specific situation. While great effort has been made to assure all information is complete and accurate as of the time this resource was issued, given the continuously evolving health care environment and the particular circumstances of individual cases, no assurance can be given that the information is entirely complete or accurate in every conceivable respect (and, as such, NHIA and its board members, committee/work group members, officers and employees disclaim all liability for the accuracy or completeness of this resource, and disclaim all warranties, express or implied to its incorrect use).

First Edition September 2023

Book design by Jamie Baylis

ISBN 978-0-9883090-5-0

Published by the National Home Infusion Association
1600 Duke Street Suite 410
Alexandra, VA 22314
www.nhia.org
Communications@NHIA.org

The Sterile Compounding Advanced Certificate Training is supported through an educational grant from **Baxter**.

Special thanks to the following organizations for sharing photographs to help illustrate this material:

- B. Braun Medical
- Contec, Inc.
- Germfree Laboratories
- New England Life Care
- Optum
- Pure Microbiology, LLC
- Yale New Haven Health System

About the National Home Infusion Association (NHIA)

NHIA is a trade association that represents companies that provide medically necessary infusion therapies to patients in alternate sites, as well as companies that manufacture and supply infusion and specialty pharmacy products. The association's mission is to provide advocacy, education, and resources to the infusion provider community so the patients they serve can lead healthy, independent lives. For more information, visit www.nhia.org.

NHIA
National Home Infusion Association

ADVANCED CERTIFICATE TRAINING

NHIA ACT

Sterile Compounding

BY ABBY ROTH, BS, CMQ/OE

Introduction and History of
Sterile Compounding Standards

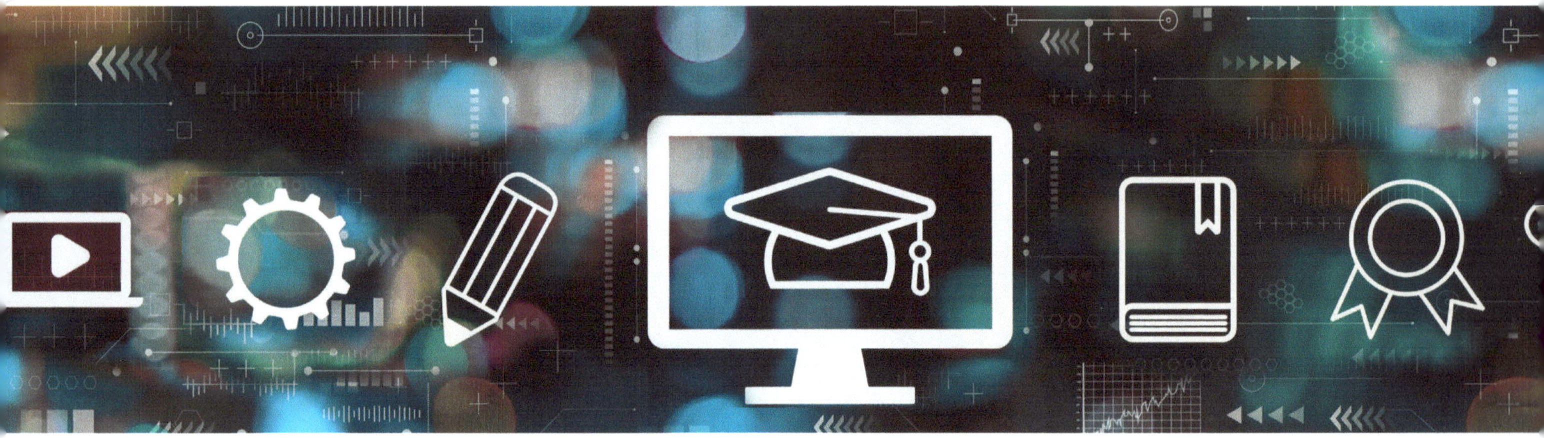

Home and alternate site infusion pharmacies are expected to provide safe and effective sterile preparations to patients receiving care in the home or other ambulatory care settings, such as ambulatory infusion suites (AIS) or long-term care facilities. Advances in drug delivery technology greatly expand the number of parenteral drugs that can be given in the home setting. This, in turn, creates a need for even greater vigilance and adherence to sterile compounding professional standards and practices.

Since the early 1990s there has been an increased interest in clean rooms, environmental monitoring, training in aseptic technique, validation of compounding personnel, and final preparation testing. Published reports of patient injury and death related to improperly compounded sterile preparations (CSPs) have prompted the reexamination of standards pertaining to aseptic practices for preparing medications intended to be sterile and the environments in which CSPs are prepared. Unfortunately, incidents involving patient injury and death due to poor technique and contaminated products still occur. The most tragic incident occurred in 2012 when a compounding pharmacy, New England Compounding Center (NECC), located in Massachusetts dispensed thousands of contaminated CSPs to 23 states, causing close to 800 patients to become ill and more than 100 deaths.[1,2] As a result, 14 individuals, including the owner and head pharmacist, were convicted on several federal criminal charges for their respective roles in producing the contaminated medicines.[3]

The NECC tragedy paved the way for significant changes to USP <797>, sterile compounding state laws, how pharmacies are inspected, and how outsourcing facilities are defined. If you are not familiar with this event, consider reading *Kill Shot* by Jason Dearen. It provides an excellent account of the patient issues, identification of the fungus responsible, and the details related to sterile compounding conditions.

USP and Compounding

Well before the NECC incident, the United States Pharmacopeial Convention (USP) was actively involved in compounding safety. In 1996, USP <1206> Sterile Drug Products for Home Use was released.[4] In the early-2000s, USP convened volunteers with extensive scientific expertise from areas of clinical practice, academia, and industry to develop clear standards for the safe compounding of sterile preparations. And, in 2004, USP published Chapter <797>, Pharmaceutical Compounding—Sterile Preparations (USP <797>), which became the first standard of practice for the preparation of all CSPs for patient use. It replaced USP Chapter <1206>. The renumbering of the revised chapter moved this information from the educational/advisory section of USP standards to the required and enforceable General Tests and Assays section.

In 2008, USP <797> was revised with the same intent but provided clarity to further help to prevent patient harm from inaccurate or contaminated CSPs. In February 2016, USP published Chapter <800> Hazardous Drugs—Handling in Healthcare Settings (USP <800>) with the purpose of providing a standard of practice for handling hazardous drugs in health care settings.

The latest revisions to USP <797> were released in 2022 and become official November 1, 2023. This revision is easier to read and more directive regarding documentation requirements and processes. The standard introduced the concept of a designated person (DP), revised how it classifies CSPs (Category 1, 2, and 3), clarified exceptions for immediate-use and preparation according to package insert, and limited the extension of beyond use dates (BUDs).

It is important to note that USP <797> and <800> are minimum standards. Facilities should strive to meet and exceed the minimum guidelines as well as additional requirements and/or best practices. While USP itself does not enforce compounding standards, <797> and <800> are potentially enforceable by a number of regulatory, accrediting, and licensing agencies. Accrediting organizations (AOs), including The Joint Commission (TJC), Accreditation Commission for Health Care (ACHC), state boards of pharmacy, and others adopt the current versions of these chapters and incorporate them into their routine survey processes. Accreditation standards require organizations to review and establish standards of practice that are aligned with both USP <797> and <800> into their policies, procedures, processes, and patient care practices when appropriate. In addition, the standards established in both USP chapters must be addressed in those states in which the state regulatory boards have partially or entirely adopted the standards.

Practical Solution: *Because standards change often and can differ depending on the issuing body, it is highly recommended that infusion providers periodically perform a gap analysis to ensure ongoing compliance with organizational standards of practice, accreditation standards, and state board of pharmacy regulations.*

Regulatory Oversight of Compounding

As a result of the NECC incident, Congress made important updates to the Federal Food, Drug, and Cosmetic Act (FD&C Act) regarding compounding for humans. Enacted on November 27, 2013, the Drug Quality and Security Act (DQSA) clarified how it defined 503A pharmacies and created a new category for large compounding facilities called 503B Outsourcing Facilities (503B). Section 503A describes conditions under which compounded human preparations are exempt from the FD&C Act under the conditions that the drugs are compounded based on a valid, patient-specific prescription among other requirements. Outsourcing facilities are subject to current Good Manufacturing Practices (cGMP) and can provide CSPs that are not identified for a particular patient. Another key difference is that a 503A compounding pharmacy falls under the purview of its state board of pharmacy, while FDA has oversight of a 503B outsourcing facility.

Over the last few years, we have seen a positive change in the number of State Boards of Pharmacy that require compliance with USP <797>. A report published in 2018 by Pew Charitable Trust found that 32 state boards of pharmacy require traditional (503A) pharmacies that compound sterile drugs for humans to be in full compliance. The study also found that an additional 11 states had strong sterile compounding requirements, with 10 of these states indicating that their practice

Exhibit 1

Comparison of USP <797> and cGMP Expectations

Feature	USP <797>	cGMP
Gloved fingertip and thumb sampling	• Every 6 months with employee competency assessment for Category 1 and 2 • Every 3 months with employee competency assessment and after each batch preparation for Category 3	With each batch during the compounding process, including testing of selected areas of the gown
Garb requirements	• Sterile gloves, non-sterile gowns, head and face coverings, and shoe covers for Category 1 and 2 • All sterile garb for Category 3	All materials must be sterile
Exposed skin	Neck, cheeks, eyes, and forehead may be exposed	No exposed skin
Surface sampling	• Monthly for Category 1 and 2 • Weekly and in the primary engineering control (PEC) at the end of each batch for Category 3	Batch-specific; in ISO* Class 5 area for every batch
Viable Air Sampling	• Every 6 months for Category 1 and 2 • Monthly for Category 3	Batch-specific; surface and air samples, viable and non-viable during compounding in ISO* Class 5 area for every batch
Use of sporicidal agents	• Monthly for Category 1 and 2 • Weekly for certain surfaces for those compounding Category 3 CSPs	Typically, weekly
Sterile cleaning agents	Only agents used in the PEC and any Isopropyl Alcohol (IPA)	All agents must be sterile
CSP is required to be patient-specific	Yes	No

*ISO-International Organization for Standardization

requirements are "equivalent or stricter" than USP <797>.[5] According to the National Association of Boards of Pharmacy (NABP) 2022 Survey of Pharmacy Law, 41 states require compliance with USP <797>. The 9 states and the District of Columbia that do not may have statutes, regulations, or policies that incorporate USP <797> requirements.[6]

Even with this progress, FDA continues to take a more direct role in the oversight of compounding activities. The agency has issued several guidance documents that limit compounding activities and give FDA the ability to inspect 503A compounders. Home infusion providers may see inspectors from FDA in their facilities in addition to accreditation and state board of pharmacy inspectors. Because of this, home infusion providers must also be familiar with the relevant FDA guidance and the cGMPs.

Exhibit 1 provides a general comparison of USP <797> and cGMP standards. Understanding the differences puts into perspective the additional quality control measures that go into providing safe medications with longer BUDs or expiration dates.

There are a number of FDA guidance documents relevant to 503A sterile compounding.

- Insanitary Conditions at Compounding Facilities
- Standard Memorandum of Understanding Addressing Certain Distributions of Compounded Drug Products Between the [insert STATE BOARD OF PHARMACY or OTHER APPROPRIATE STATE AGENCY] and the U.S. Food and Drug Administration
- Hospital and Health System Compounding Under Section 503A of the Federal Food, Drug, and Cosmetic Act
- Pharmacy Compounding of Human Drug Products Under Section 503A of the Federal Food, Drug, and Cosmetic Act Guidance (PDF - 86KB) List of Bulk Drug Substances that can be used to Compound Drug Products in Accordance with Section 503A the Federal Food, Drug, and Cosmetic Act
- Amendments to the List of Bulk Drug Substances that can be used to Compound Drug Products in Accordance with Section 503A of the Federal Food, Drug, and Cosmetic Act
- Compounded Drug Products That Are Essentially Copies of a Commercially Available Drug Product Under Section 503A of the Federal Food, Drug, and Cosmetic Act

Compounding Timeline

1971 National Coordinating Committee Large Volume Parenterals (NCCLVP) is founded to address problems with microbial contamination and other issues[7]

1975 **1976** **1977** **1978** **1979** **1980**

NCCLVP publishes recommendations[8]

1992 ASHP Technical Assistance Bulletin, "Quality Assurance for Pharmacy Prepared Products" and USP proposed <1074> Dispensing Practices for Sterile Drug Products Intended for Home Use are released in an effort for pharmacists to take responsibility for ensuring proper preparation, labeling, storage, dispensing, and delivery of CSPs.[4,9] Lack of enforcement and financial support did little for the implementation of these recommendations.

1996 USP <1206> Sterile Drug Products for Home Use is released.[4]

1998 The US Food and Drug Administration Modernization Act (FDAMA) of 1997 is signed into law. Section 503A, titled "Pharmacy Compounding," defined the scope of compounding and sought to protect patients from the unnecessary use of extemporaneously compounded drugs and gave FDA the ability to determine which drugs that if compounded could adversely affect safety or effectiveness.[9]

2001 The Supreme Court ruled the soliciting and advertising provisions in section 503A unconstitutional, leaving a void of federal regulation for pharmacy and the FDA.[9]

2004 USP <797> Pharmaceutical Compounding—Sterile Preparations becomes official.

2008 A revision to USP <797> Pharmaceutical Compounding—Sterile Preparations is released.

2012 The NECC CSP contamination incident resulted in nearly 800 affected patients and more than 100 deaths across 23 states.[1,2]

2013 The Drug Quality and Security Act (DQSA) clarified how it defines 503A pharmacies and created a new category for large compounding facilities called 503B Outsourcing Facilities (503B).

2016 USP General Chapter <800> Hazardous Drugs—Handling in Healthcare Settings is released.

2022 A revision to USP <797> Pharmaceutical Compounding—Sterile Preparations is released.

References

1. Raymond, N. Pharmacist in deadly U.S. meningitis outbreak resentenced to 10-1/2 years in prison. Reuters. July 21, 2021.
2. McCune, G. Meningitis outbreak expands to 15 states with Pennsylvania case. Reuters. October 15, 2012.
3. The United States Department of Justice. 14 Indicted in Connection with New England Compounding Center and Nationwide Fungal Meningitis Outbreak. December 14, 2017.
4. Ashworth, L. The USP and Compounding Sterile Medications. *Association of Portuguese Hospital Pharmacists.* November 21, 2015.
5. The Pew Charitable Trusts. State Oversight of Drug Compounding. February 26, 2018.
6. National Association of Boards of Pharmacy. 2022 Survey of Pharmacy Law. 2021.
7. Barker, K. Interim Report National Coordinating Committee on large Volume Parenterals. *Drug Intelligence & Clinical Pharmacy,* Volume: 7 issue: 10, page(s): 475-477. October 1, 1973
8. American Society of Health-System Pharmacists. *ASHP Guidelines on Compounding Sterile Preparations.* 2014.
9. American Society of Health-System Pharmacists. *The ASHP Discussion Guide on USP Chapter <797>for Compounding Sterile Preparations.* 2013

UNIT 1

Definitions and Scope of the United States Pharmacopeia (USP) Standards

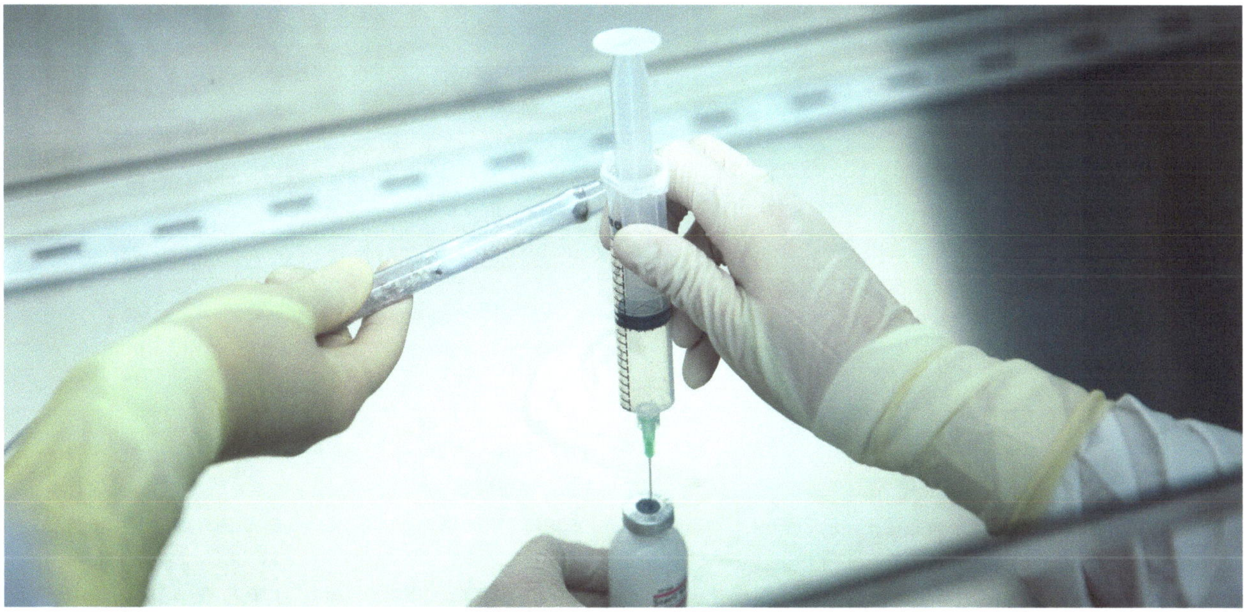

Photo courtesy of Contec, Inc.

Proper compounding technique is critical to the safe preparation of sterile medications. A smoke source can be used to identify the blocking of first air to the critical site, as shown in the image above.

The first section of USP General Chapter <797> is titled "Introduction and Scope." It describes the purpose of the chapter and identifies how the chapter applies to the different compounding acts. Provisions and exemptions to following the chapter are also defined. This unit reviews important definitions related to sterile compounding and identifies the scope of USP General Chapter <797> so that readers may better understand how the chapter applies to their sterile compounding operation.

Differentiating Compounded Preparations from Aseptically Prepared Products

How do you define compounding? Which compounding acts are included in your definition?

There is no single definition of compounding. The statutory definition of compounding found in 21 U.S. Code § 353a is a negative one in the sense that it defines compounding by what it is not. It states:

> *". . . the term 'compounding' does not include mixing, reconstituting, or other such acts that are performed in accordance with directions contained in approved labeling provided by the product's manufacturer and other manufacturer directions consistent with that labeling."*[1]

In simple terms, the FDA views drugs as either: 1) FDA-approved through the New Drug Application (NDA) process, or 2) compounds. After the New England Compounding Center (NECC) incident in 2012, the FDA sought to extend its authority over compounding and expanded on the definition slightly through the Drug Quality and Security Act (DQSA). The DQSA refers to compounding more broadly by encompassing a variety of manipulations that may result in "altering" a substance to create a drug. From the DQSA:

> *"The term 'compounding' includes the combining, admixing, mixing, diluting, pooling, reconstituting, or otherwise altering of a drug or bulk drug substance to create a drug."*[2]

The USP <797> definition aligns more closely with the DQSA, offers limited distinction between aseptically prepared approved drugs and compounded preparations and includes repackaging in the definition of compounding. Under the FDA, repackaging is not considered compounding and falls under different guidance. USP <797> defines compounding as:

> *"The process of combining, admixing, diluting, pooling, reconstituting, repackaging, or otherwise altering a drug or bulk drug substance to create a sterile medication."*[3]

Notice the word sterile is included in this definition. Remember, USP <797> is strictly for the preparation of sterile medications. The previous definitions listed are for the general term of compounding. Sterility would apply based on the intended medication prepared.

Eliminating the Confusion

The term "aseptically prepared products" (APPs) does not appear in USP <797> or other regulatory documents. But it is a clear and understandable way to distinguish between commercially available FDA-approved drug products that require aseptic preparation from compounded sterile preparations (CSPs). This distinction is important for compliance with FDA guidance, however it is critical that both types of preparations are made according to nationally accepted standards for 503A pharmacies. **USP <797> standards should be applied when preparing both APPs and CSPs.**

Ascepticaly Prepared Product (APP)

- A commercially available FDA-approved drug product that requires aseptic preparation in accordance with the product labeling

Compounded Sterile Preparation (CSP)[3]

- A preparation intended to be sterile that is created by combining, admixing, diluting, pooling, reconstituting, repackaging, or otherwise altering a drug product or bulk drug

Home and alternate site infusion providers engage in activities involving the manipulation of drugs, which are usually FDA approved, sterile, and conventionally manufactured to create finished dosage forms to be infused to the patient. Some preparations made by home infusion providers would be considered non-compounded preparations by the FDA because they are prepared doses of an FDA-approved drug. These products could be differentiated by referring to them as "aseptically prepared products." Other preparations, such as parenteral nutrition would clearly meet the definition of a compounded preparation. By USP standards, most of the preparations made by home infusion providers would be considered compounded preparations.

Regardless of the technical definitions, home infusion providers have embraced the USP compounding standards because many of the preparations they make will be stored by the patient for several days before being infused, and longer storage times increase the risk for microbial growth. For purposes of this module, the term "compounded sterile preparations" or CSPs, will refer generally to parenteral nutrition, preparations made from active pharmaceutical ingredients, or preparations that combine 2 or more FDA-approved drugs (other than diluents). Aseptically prepared products (APPs) refer to making finished dosage forms of FDA-approved drugs.

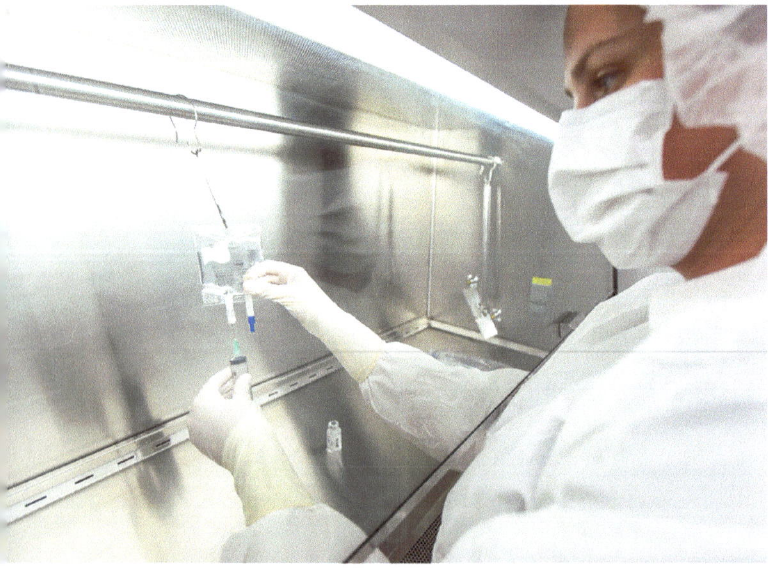

Photo courtesy of Contec, Inc.

Application of USP Standards

The objective of USP <797> is to establish a standard for the prevention of patient harm from preparations that are:[3]

1. Contaminated
2. Contain excessive bacterial endotoxins
3. Vary from the intended strength of correct ingredients
4. Have chemical and physical incompatibilities or contaminants
5. Made from ingredients of inappropriate quality

Have you ever stopped to think about how the CSPs you prepare could affect someone's life?

Obviously, these medications can ease pain, provide nutrition, or stop a harmful infection. But what if they are improperly prepared? What if the wrong drug was used or they are contaminated with microorganisms? These mistakes can be life altering to a patient and their family. What if it was your family? How would you feel? Use that feeling to fuel your dedication to the safe preparation of APPs and CSPs.

Recognizing that direct contact with non-sterile surfaces is the principal source of contamination, the requirements set forth by USP apply to all personnel who prepare sterile medications as well as all places where APPs and CSPs are prepared. Aseptic technique principals must be adhered to when preparing any medication intended to be sterile. Procedures must be in place to minimize the potential for contact with non-sterile surfaces, introduction of particulate matter or biological fluids, and errors with other products.

Compliance with USP standards involves developing comprehensive policies and standard operating procedures (SOPs) for all aspects of the aseptic process, from the facility where preparations are made, to personnel training, to storage during delivery.

However, assuring compliance is the responsibility of regulatory bodies, as USP has no enforcement abilities. State boards of pharmacy and accreditation or credentialing organizations may—and do—adopt and enforce USP standards.

Understanding the Scope of USP <797>

As was previously mentioned, the goal of the chapter is to prevent patient harm. As part of this, sterility of the CSPs is essential. USP <797> provides a list of CSPs that must be sterile, which includes:[3]

- Injections, including infusions
- Irrigations for internal body cavities (This is any space that does not normally communicate with the outside of the body, such as the bladder cavity or peritoneal cavity. Irrigations for the mouth, rectal cavity, and sinus cavity are not required to be sterile.)
- Ophthalmic dosage forms
- Aqueous preparations for pulmonary inhalation (Nasal dosage forms intended for local application are not required to be sterile.)
- Baths and soaks for live organs and tissues
- Implants

There are a few specific practices that the chapter defines as part of its scope (see Exhibit 1 for clarification). Not all of these will affect what pharmacies prepare for home infusion patients, but it is interesting to see how the chapter applies to other preparations and activities.

Administration

There are situations when compounders are exempt from following USP <797> standards. The first situation relates to the administration of CSPs. Administration is defined as *"the direct application of a sterile product or preparation to a single patient by injecting, infusing, or otherwise providing a medication in its final form."*[3] USP Chapter <797> applies to the processes associated with preparing and storing a sterile medication right up to the time it is administered. **Administration is outside the scope of USP <797> and nothing in the standard should be interpreted to limit the time over which a sterile medication is administered to a patient.** Clinicians should, however, consider administration time when developing beyond use dates (BUDs) specifically related to the stability of the preparation

Exhibit 1

Specific Practices That Are Beyond the Scope of USP General Chapter

Repackaging	Repackaging of a sterile product or preparation from its original container into another container must be done in accordance with the chapter.
Allergenic extracts	Section 21 of USP <797> describes the standards for compounding allergenic extracts. These standards are only applicable when: • Compounding involves transfer via sterile needles and syringes of conventionally manufactured sterile allergen products and appropriate conventionally manufactured sterile added substances • Manipulations are limited to penetrating stoppers on vials with sterile needles and syringes, and transferring sterile liquids in sterile syringes to sterile vials
Hazardous drugs	Any handling of hazardous drugs must comply with USP General Chapter <800> Hazardous Drugs — Handling in Healthcare Settings.
Blood-derived and other biological materials	If compounding requires the manipulation of a patient's blood-derived or other biological material: • Manipulations must be separated from other compounding activities and equipment • Cross-contamination procedures must be implemented and included in standard operating procedures (SOPs)
Sterile radio-pharmaceuticals	The preparation of radiopharmaceuticals is outside the scope of USP <797> and is subject to the requirements in USP <825> Radiopharmaceuticals — Preparation, Compounding, Dispensing, and Repackaging

Immediate-Use CSPs

A second exemption allows for provisions for compounding to occur outside of a clean room suite or segregated compounding area (SCA). This lack of control may seem unsafe, but the chapter requires several conditions to be met to ensure access to certain compounded medications where the risk of harm is low. The initial exemption for immediate-use appeared in the 2008 version of <797> and was limited to emergency situations or when the product required immediate administration—within 1 hour of preparation. To qualify for this exemption, the process could not involve more than 3 original containers, could have no more than 2 entries into any single container, and had to be a continuous preparation process not lasting more than 1 hour. The immediate-use exemption from the 2008 chapter did not apply to hazardous drugs.[4]

Immediate-use CPS are no longer limited to emergency situations. This allows for better patient access to medication. The immediate-use exemption allows for up to 3 unique components (regardless of the number of original vials or containers) without complying with USP standards if there is evidence supporting the physical and chemical compatibility. Additionally, the administration must occur within 4 hours of the start of preparation. This exemption is limited to preparing single or multiple doses for a single patient. If single-dose vials are used, any unused portion must be discarded and cannot be used to compound additional preparations. Exhibit 2 outlines all applicable USP <797> immediate-use CSP exemptions.

Preparation According to Approved Labeling

USP <797> provides flexibility for aseptically preparing doses of FDA-approved drugs according to the manufacturer's labeling. Remember, the preparation of an FDA-approved drug according to the approved instructions is not considered compounding per the statutory definition, therefore, USP allows for mixing and reconstituting preparations in accordance with

Exhibit 2

Compounding Exemptions from USP General Chapter <797>[5]

Exemption	Criteria for Being Exempt from USP Requirements
Immediate and direct administration	• Aseptic processes are followed and written SOPs are in place • Personnel are trained and demonstrate competency related to the tasks performed • Evidence supporting chemical and physical compatibility is available • No more than 3 different sterile products (components, not containers) are used • Preparation is for a single patient (not prepared in batches) • Administration begins within 4 hours of the start of preparation • Unused drug from single-dose containers is discarded after compounding is complete • Unless administered by the preparer or administration is witnessed by the preparer, the CSP is labeled with the names and amounts of all active ingredients, the name of the preparer, and the exact 4-hour timeframe within which the administration is performed

Preparing a CSP according to the package labeling	• Mixing, reconstitution, or other such acts occur in accordance with the preparation instructions as described on the FDA-approved labeling
	• The labeling information includes specific information regarding:
	  ○ Diluent to be used
	  ○ Final strength
	  ○ Storage time
	  ○ Container closure system
	• The starting components are conventionally manufactured sterile products
	• Prepared as a single dose for an individual patient

Docking and activation with proprietary bag and vial systems	• In accordance with labeling • For immediate administration to an individual patient

Administration is outside the scope of USP <797> and nothing in the standard should be interpreted to limit the time over which a sterile medication is administered to a patient.

the label without complying with USP standards. This exemption limits the process to preparing a single dose of a sterile medication for an individual patient, and to those products whose approved labeling includes information for the diluent, resultant strength, container closure system, and storage time.[3]

Proprietary Bag and Vial Systems

USP <797> also addresses the docking and activation of proprietary bag and vial systems such as, addEASE®, ADD-Vantage™, and Mini Bag Plus. If these systems are docked and activated for immediate administration to an individual patient, it is not considered compounding and is exempt from the requirements of USP <797>. However, the systems are not always used as originally intended. When the proprietary bag and vial systems are docked and stored for future activation and administration, the aseptic procedures used in the preparations must be performed in accordance with all requirements of USP <797>.

Open to Advancements

Technology and techniques related to compounding are always evolving. To ensure <797> is inclusive of new advancements, there is a section that discusses how to incorporate them into your processes. For a technology, technique, material, or procedure other than those described in the chapter to be implemented it must not be:

> *"inferior to those described in the chapter and be validated for the intended purpose."*

Summary

The act of sterile compounding has many facets and the medications prepared come with different risks. Some of these acts fall under the purview of USP <797>, while others are outside the scope of the standard. As someone who oversees or performs sterile compounding, it is important to recognize what is and what is not defined as compounding and to understand how the regulations apply. This insight ensures medications are prepared safely.

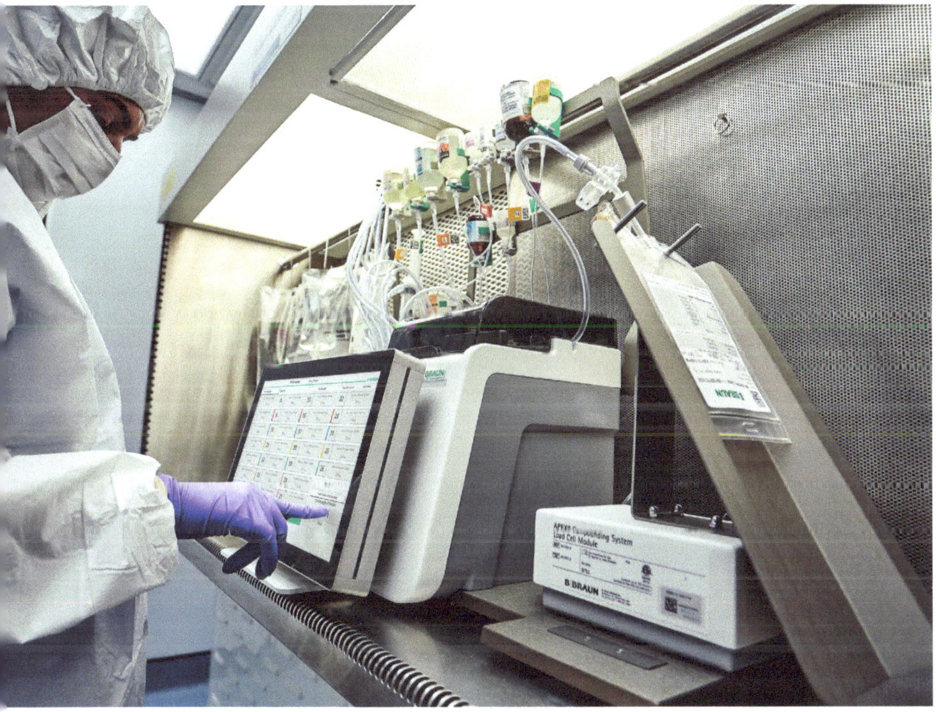

Photo courtesy of B. Braun Medical

References

1. United States Code, 2006 Edition, Supplement 5, Title 21 - FOOD AND DRUGS. CHAPTER 9 - FEDERAL FOOD, DRUG, AND COSMETIC ACT SUBCHAPTER V - DRUGS AND DEVICES Part A - Drugs and Devices Sec. 353a - Pharmacy compounding. 2011
2. Drug Quality and Security Act. Compounding Quality Act. Title 1-Drug Compounding. 2013.
3. United States Pharmacopeia. <797> Pharmaceutical Compounding Sterile Preparations. Revision. November 2022.
4. United States Pharmacopeia. <797> Pharmaceutical Compounding—Sterile Preparations. Proposed Revision. 2008.
5. Sullivan, C. The Revised USP Sterile Compounding Standards: Implications for Home Infusion and Alternate Site Providers; INFUSION Magazine July/August 2019

Summary: Definitions and Scope of USP

Defining Compounding

21 U.S. Code § 353a	*"...the term 'compounding' does not include mixing, reconstituting, or other such acts that are performed in accordance with directions contained in approved labeling provided by the product's manufacturer and other manufacturer directions consistent with that labeling."*[1]
DQSA	*"The term 'compounding' includes the combining, admixing, mixing, diluting, pooling, reconstituting, or otherwise altering of a drug or bulk drug substance to create a drug."*[2]
USP <797>	*"The process of combining, admixing, diluting, pooling, reconstituting, repackaging, or otherwise altering a drug or bulk drug substance to create a sterile medication."*[3]

Overview of the Scope of USP General Chapter <797>

Who	USP requirements apply to all personnel who prepare sterile medications and all places were APPs and CSPs are prepared
What	CSPs that must be sterile include, but are not limited to: • Injections, including infusions • Irrigations for internal body cavities • Ophthalmic dosage forms • Aqueous preparations for pulmonary inhalation • Baths and soaks for live organs and tissues • Implants
Where	USP requirements apply to all places were APPs and CSPs are prepared
When	USP requirements apply whenever CSPs are prepared, unless specified in the chapter. The following are beyond the scope of the chapter if the specified provisions are met: 1. Administration 2. Immediate-use CSPs 3. Preparation according to approved labeling 4. Proprietary bag and vial systems
Why	The objective of USP <797> is to establish a standard for the prevention of patient harm from aseptically prepared or compounded preparations that are:[3] 1. Contaminated 2. Contain excessive bacterial endotoxins 3. Vary from the intended strength of correct ingredients 4. Have chemical and physical incompatibilities or contaminants made from ingredients of inappropriate quality

Compounding Exemptions from USP General Chapter <797>[4]

Exemption	Criteria for Being Exempt from USP Requirements
Immediate and direct administration	• Aseptic processes are followed and written SOPs are in place • Personnel are trained and demonstrate competency related to the tasks performed • Evidence supporting chemical and physical compatibility is available • No more than 3 different sterile products (components, not containers) are used • Preparation is for a single patient (not prepared in batches) • Administration begins within 4 hours of the start of preparation • Unused drug from single-dose containers is discarded after compounding is complete • Unless administered by the preparer or administration is witnessed by the preparer, the CSP is labeled with the names and amounts of all active ingredients, the name of the preparer, and the exact 4-hour timeframe within which the administration is performed

Preparing a CSP according to the package labeling	• Mixing, reconstitution, or other such acts occur in accordance with the preparation instructions as described on the FDA-approved labeling
	• The labeling information includes specific information regarding:
	  ○ Diluent to be used
	  ○ Final strength
	  ○ Storage time
	  ○ Container closure system
	• The starting components are conventionally manufactured sterile products
	• Prepared as a single dose for an individual patient

Docking and activation with proprietary bag and vial systems	• In accordance with labeling • For immediate administration to an individual patient

References

1. United States Code, 2006 Edition, Supplement 5, Title 21 - FOOD AND DRUGS. CHAPTER 9 - FEDERAL FOOD, DRUG, AND COSMETIC ACT SUBCHAPTER V - DRUGS AND DEVICES Part A - Drugs and Devices Sec. 353a - Pharmacy compounding. 2011
2. Drug Quality and Security Act. Compounding Quality Act. Title I-Drug Compounding. 2013.
3. United States Pharmacopeia. <797> Pharmaceutical Compounding—Sterile Preparations. Revision. November 2022.
4. Sullivan, C. The Revised USP Sterile Compounding Standards: Implications for Home Infusion and Alternate Site Providers; INFUSION Magazine July/August 2019

UNIT 2

Categories of Compounded Sterile Preparations (CSPs) and Beyond Use Dates (BUDs)

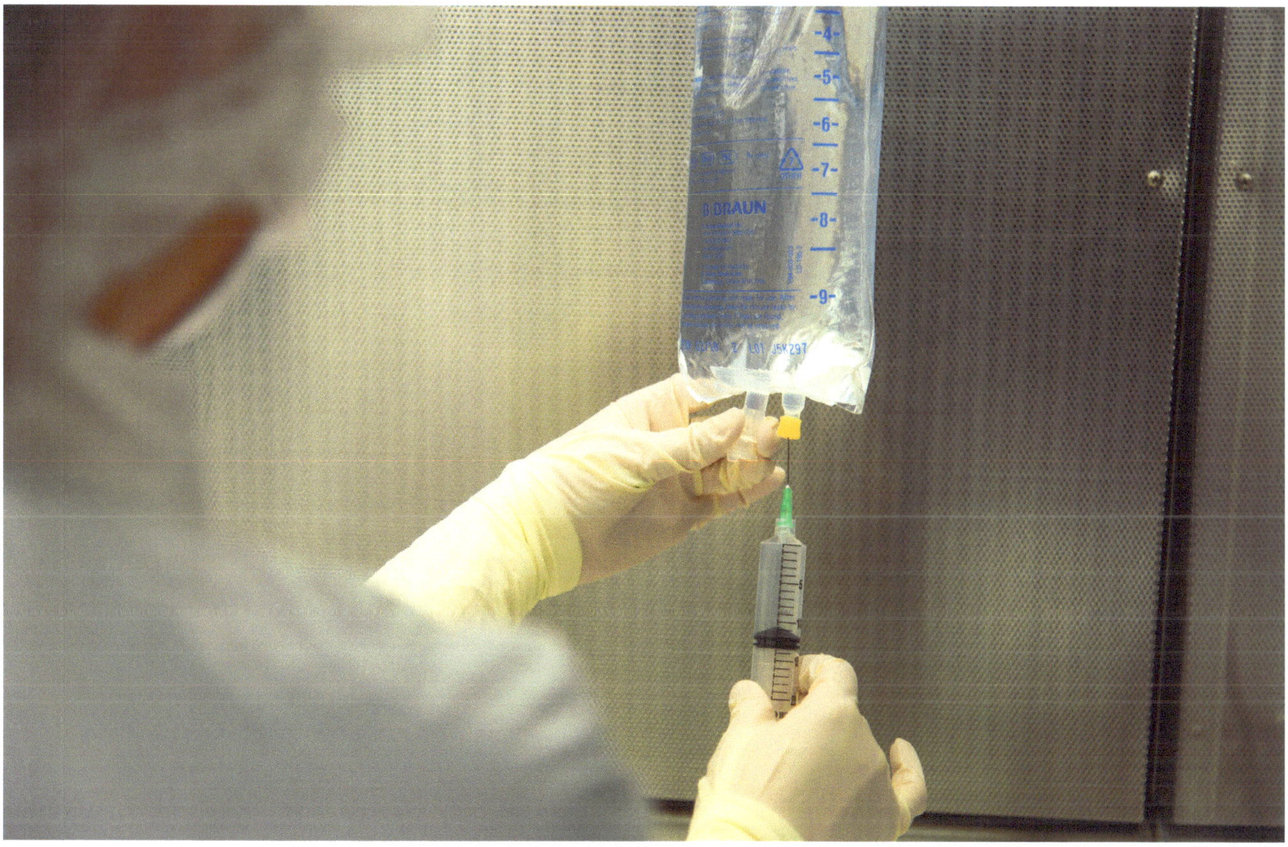

Photo courtesy of Contec, Inc.

For many years, CSPs fell into essentially 4 categories: low-risk with 12-hour beyond use date (BUD), low-risk, medium-risk, and high-risk. The categories focused mainly on the components used and number of punctures into a vial, bag, etc. Through the revision process, USP General Chapter <797> has shifted from this paradigm to one that focuses on where the CSP was prepared, with BUDs based on whether certain testing is performed. This unit will explore the compounding categories and review the BUDs that can be assigned, based on USP requirements.

Why Compounding Categories?

The process for assessing and determining the risk for contamination, poor quality, and errors associated with the preparation of sterile medications has evolved since USP <797> was introduced in 2004. In the 2008 version, CSPs were categorized as either low-, medium-, or high-risk. The preparer assigned a level of risk to the final preparation based on the complexity of the aseptic process, the number and type of ingredients used, and various other factors. However, many experts argued this method of classification was flawed because it could inappropriately infer confidence in a preparation's quality. For example, a product designated as "low-risk" still has potential for contamination if the environment, technique, or ingredients were of poor quality. Likewise, a high-risk, terminally sterilized CSP prepared under well-controlled conditions and tested for sterility is unlikely to cause harm. For these reasons, the 2023 revision introduced a new classification system to describe the likelihood of contamination of a CSP more objectively.

This new system has 3 categories, which are identified as Category 1, Category 2, and Category 3.[1] According to USP, *"this change was proposed to avoid inaccurately conferring a level of risk to a particular CSP without consideration for all factors that influence the quality of that CSP."*[2] The chosen naming system is neutral and does not specifically define a level of risk. Instead, the

BUDs vs. Expiration Dates

There is quite a bit of confusion surrounding the terms BUD and expiration date. It's important to know the difference and how they both apply to a sterile compounding operation.

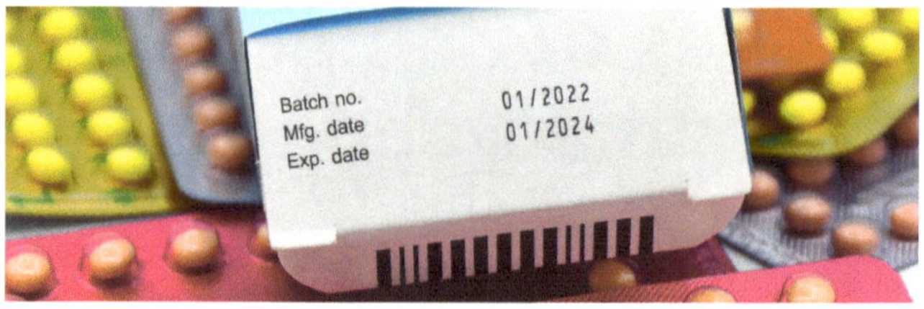

BUD[1]	Expiration Date[1]
• Either the date, or hour and date, after which a CSP must not be used.	• The time during which a product can be expected to meet the requirements of the USP-NF monograph, if one exists, or maintain expected quality provided it is kept under the specified storage conditions.
• Applies to all CSPs	• Applies to all conventionally manufactured products, active pharmaceutical ingredients (APIs), and added substances

category is distinguished primarily by the conditions under which the CSP is made and the timeframe within which it is used.

In developing the compounding categories, USP considered the:[2]

1. Need for a scientifically robust and risk-based approach to assigning BUDs, including both stability and sterility considerations
2. Balance of patient access to cost-effective CSPs with rigorous quality standards
3. Cost of implementing these categories in different practice settings
4. Implications on regulatory oversight and enforcement for the requirements

Categories and BUDs are Intertwined

Each CSP must be assigned a BUD, which is the date or the hour and date beyond which the preparation must not be used and must be discarded. It is determined from the date and time that the preparation of the CSP is initiated.[1] Once the BUD has passed, the CSP must be discarded.

When reading the BUD definition, the word "used" may have stood out and leave one asking how "used" is defined. Used means the moment the medication is given to the patient but does not include the time over which the CSP is administered. Essentially, administration of the CSP must start before the BUD is reached.
This distinction is important because the length of administration must be considered when determining the BUD for a CSP in this setting. In home infusion, CSPs may be administered over long periods of time at room temperature using infusion pumps; therefore, ensuring the preparation integrity and stability throughout its administration is important for patient safety and efficacy.

Practical Solution: *Stability is* "the extent to which a product or preparation retains physical and chemical properties and characteristics within specified limits throughout its expiration or BUD." *This is essentially stating that the CSP prepared needs to work as expected through its BUD. Therefore, home and alternate site infusion providers need to consider this efficacy through the administration time. Evidence-based information must be used when identifying the stability of a drug. This information can come from:*

- *FDA-approved labeling from the drug manufacturer*
- *Your own stability studies*
- *Written communication from the drug manufacturer*
- *Stability data published in the literature*

The BUD that can be assigned to a CSP is based on the category by which it was prepared. Remember, the categories are designed based on microbial risk to the CSP. Let's look at how BUDs and the categories are related.

CSP Categories and Their BUDs

Do you know which CSP categories are compounded at your organization? What are the BUDs that can be assigned? Which quality measures have you implemented based on the categories you compound?

USP <797> describes 3 categories of CSPs; Category 1, Category 2, and Category 3. Rather than leaving it to the preparer to confer a level of risk to a CSP, the classification is based on the conditions under which the CSP is made. The differentiation between Category 1 and Categories 2 and 3 is the placement of the primary engineering control (PEC). Category 2 can be differentiated from Category 3 by the additional sterile processing requirements that are implemented, such as sterile garb and increased viable sampling frequencies.

Category 1, 2, and 3 CSPs can be compounded by using only sterile starting ingredients or by using some or all non-sterile ingredients. If non-sterile ingredients or tools are used, the sterility of the preparation must be achieved through a sterilization process. If all sterile ingredients are used, the sterility of these preparations must not be compromised during the compounding process.

Category 1 refers to CSPs prepared in a primary engineering control (PEC) that is placed in an unclassified area (no anteroom or buffer room). This type of arrangement is referred to as a segregated compounding area (SCA).

Exhibit 1

Category 1 Beyond Use Dates[1]

Storage Conditions	
Controlled Room Temperature (20-25°C)	Refrigerator (2-8°C)
BUD: ≤ 12 hours	*BUD:* ≤ 24 hours

Category 1 CSPs can include hazardous CSPs and non-sterile to sterile preparations. BUDs for Category 1 CSPs are short (see Exhibit 1) and do not support home infusion protocols, which require the ability to store the CSP for several days.

Category 2 CSPs are made inside a PEC placed within an ISO classified buffer room, which is served by an ISO classified anteroom. Category 2 CSPs allow for longer BUDs which are based on the following:

- The compounding process
- Was the preparation aseptically prepared or terminally sterilized?
- Were the ingredients and equipment used sterile or non-sterile?
- Release testing
- Was sterility and endotoxin testing performed?
- Environmental conditions
- What was the temperature of storage?

Important BUD Notes

1. Some BUDs are in hours while some are listed in days.
2. The BUDs in the category tables are based on risk to the sterility of the CSP. This lack of sterility assurance could be from microbial contamination or not achieving and maintaining sterility.
3. Evaluate the formulation to ensure the CSP will remain chemically and physically stable through the BUD and required administration time.
4. The CSPs packaging must maintain its integrity for the duration of the BUD.
5. The BUD equals the shortest of the drugs' chemical stability or the microbial limit determined by the category table.

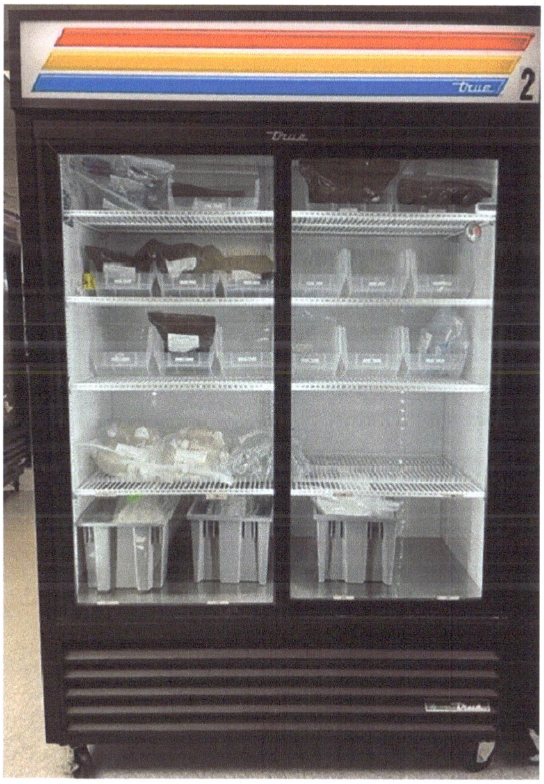

Photo courtesy of New England Life Care

The Category 2 and 3 BUD tables list 2 compounding methods: aseptically processed CSPs and terminally sterilized CSPs. USP <797> clearly defines the difference in these 2 methods.

Aseptic processing

- Separate, sterile components are brought together under conditions that maintain their sterility.[1]
- Start with sterile, end with sterile.

OR

- Nonsterile ingredients are used to prepare a medication and sterilization is performed by filtration.
- Start with non-sterile, use a sterilizing filter, end with sterile.

Terminal sterilization

- A lethal process to sealed containers, such as dry heat, steam, or irradaition, for the purpose of achieving a probability of less than 1 in 1 million of a non-sterile unit.[1]
- Start with sterile or non-sterile, use a sterilization technology, end with sterile.

Exhibit 2 illustrates that BUDs for Category 2 CSPs can range from 1 to 90 days. There are many options for establishing the BUD, but it will start with the establishment of the components used during the compounding process to make the final determination. A large majority of the compounding taking place in home infusion falls into Category 2, which involves aseptic processing of sterile starting components. The most common maximum BUDs in home infusion include: 4 days at room temperature, 10 days refrigerated, and up to 45 days frozen. Most home infusion providers do not perform sterility testing or use terminal sterilization to extend BUDs.

Based on these USP definitions, an aseptically prepared CSP is either prepared from sterile components or prepared from non-sterile components

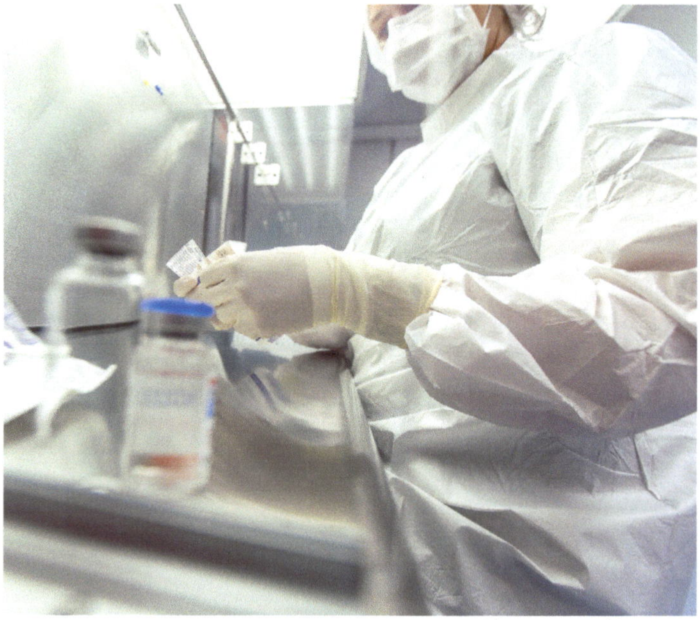

Photo courtesy of Contec, Inc.

Exhibit 2

Category 2 BUDs[1]

Preparation Details		Storage Conditions		
Compounding method	Sterility testing performed and passed	Controlled room temperature (20 – 25° C or 68 – 77° F)	Refrigerated (2 – 8° C or 36 – 46° F)	Frozen (-25 – -10° C or -13 – 14° F)
Aseptically processed CSPs	No	Prepared from 1 or more non-sterile starting component(s): 1 day	Prepared from 1 or more non-sterile starting component(s): 4 days	Prepared from 1 or more non-sterile starting component(s): 45 days
		Prepared from only sterile starting components: 4 days	Prepared from only sterile starting components: 10 days	Prepared from only sterile starting components: 45 days
	Yes	30 days	45 days	60 days
Terminally sterilized CSPs	No	14 days	28 days	45 days
	Yes	45 days	60 days	90 days

and sterilized using a 0.22-micron filter. Terminally sterilized CSPs include compounding with sterile or non-sterile starting ingredients and subsequent sterilization that includes dry heat, steam, or irradiation.

Category 3 CSPs are prepared in the same environment as Category 2 CSPs but have additional requirements for:

- Personnel qualification
- Garb
- Cleaning and disinfection
- Viable sampling
- Stability determination

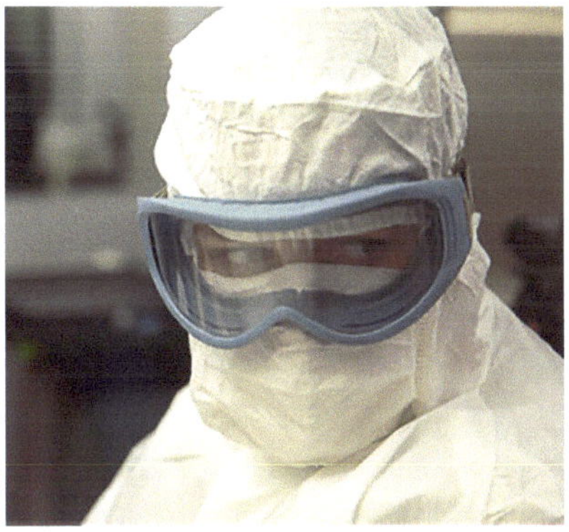

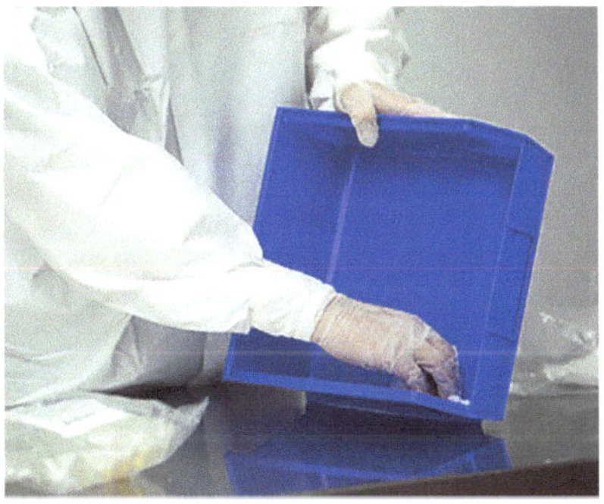

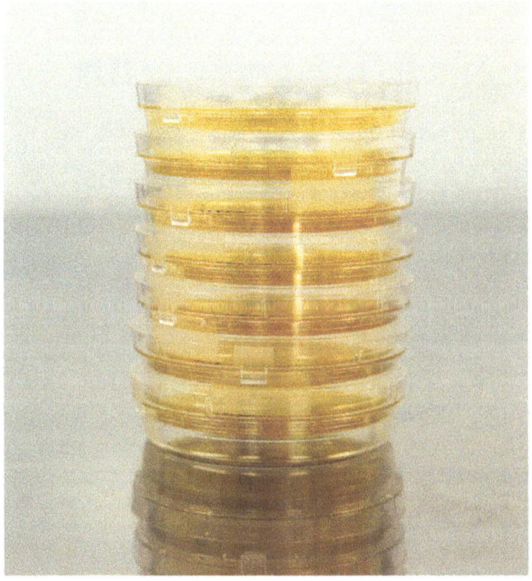

Photos courtesy of Contec, Inc.

If all these requirements are met, and sterility testing is performed, supplemented with appropriate endotoxin testing, longer BUDs than those for Category 2 CSPs may be applied, but they are limited to those indicated in the chapter. **This means that even if your organization has stability data longer than the dating in the chapter, you cannot extend the BUD based on the stability data.**

Let's examine the additional requirements for Category 3 CSPs in more detail.

Facility and Personnel Related[1]

- Personnel who compound or oversee the compounding of Category 3 CPSs must meet the additional competency requirements for hand hygiene and garbing and aseptic manipulation.
- Personnel who enter the buffer room where Category 3 CSPs are compounded, must follow the Category 3 garbing requirements regardless of whether Category 3 CSPs are prepared that day.
- Increased environmental monitoring requirements apply to all classified areas where Category 3 CSPs are compounded, regardless of Category 3 compounding frequency.
- The application frequency of sporicidal disinfectants applies to all classified areas where Category 3 CSPs are compounded.

Formulation and Testing Related[1]

- The BUD assigned to a Category 3 CSP must be supported by stability data obtained using a stability-indicating analytical method that is able to distinguish the active ingredient from its degradants and impurities (e.g., by forced degradation studies) and quantify the amount of the active ingredient.
- The Category 3 CSP must be prepared according to the exact formulation (API and other ingredients of identical grade and procedures) from which the stability data are derived.
- The Category 3 CSP must be packaged and stored in a container closure of the same materials of composition as that used in the study.
- The analytical method must be validated based on characteristics such as those described in Chapter <1225> Validation of Compendial Procedure.
- The compounding facility must have documentation of the stability study, including a description of the methodology (e.g., number of samples taken, storage conditions), validation of the method, the stability-indicating analytical method, and the results.

Exhibit 3

Category 3 BUDs[1]

Preparation and Testing Conditions	Storage Conditions		
	Controlled room temperature (20 – 25° C or 68 – 77° F)	Refrigerated (2 – 8° C or 36 – 46 F)	Frozen (-25 – -10° C or -13 – 14° F)
Aseptically processed CSPs, sterility tested, and passing all applicable tests for Category 3 CSPs	60 days	90 days	120 days
Terminally sterilized CSPs, sterility tested, and passing all applicable tests for Category 3 CSPs	90 days	120 days	180 days

- Each time the Category 3 CSP is prepared, it is sterility tested in accordance with Chapter <71> Sterility Tests, or a validated alternative method that is not inferior to <71> testing, with acceptable results.
- Each time the Category 3 CSP is prepared, it is tested for endotoxins for acceptable results, if endotoxin testing is required.

Exhibit 3 outlines the longest permitted BUDs for Category 3 CSPs.

Considerations In Assigning BUDs

Stability Considerations

In determining an appropriate BUD, one must consider both the stability and sterility of the final preparation. Stability refers to the extent to which a preparation retains physical and chemical properties and characteristics throughout its BUD and possibly through administration. Sterility is the absence of microorganisms.

Home and alternate site infusion professionals must consider which factors may affect stability, including but not exclusive to:

- Chemical and physical properties of the drug and/or its formulation
- Compatibility of the drug with the container and administration sets
- Compatibility of the drug with other components such as diluents
- Storage conditions of the final preparation

Stability data is usually derived from the FDA-approved product labeling; however, home infusion providers often use alternative containers such as elastomeric devices and syringes to hold CSPs. When using an alternative container for the CSP, the stability data may be obtained from references or studies performed by entities other than the drug manufacturer. The quality of these studies can vary, and data used from these sources must be carefully reviewed to ensure applicability. Extrapolations can be performed in some instances. For example, if a stability study shows compatibility for a container at 2 specific concentrations of a drug, then the compounder may apply those finding to any concentration falling within the study range.

Following Category 3 Requirements:
Are you thinking about compounding Category 3 CSPs occasionally? You may want to think again. USP <797> requires that any of the activities necessary to the compounding of Category 3 CSPs be performed always and not just on days when Category 3 CSPs are prepared. This ensures that the expected state of control is achieved and maintained. But it may be more than you want to maintain for an occasional CSP needing a longer BUD.

Reassigning BUDs When Changing Storage Conditions

The storage time for a CSP cannot exceed the original BUD placed on the label, and BUDs are never additive. For example (Exhibit 4), an aseptically prepared CSP using at least 1 non-sterile starting component cannot be stored for 45 days frozen, 4 days refrigerated, and 1 day at room temperature. This would be 50

Exhibit 4

Example of Proper vs. Improper Application of BUDs

Improper	45 days frozen +	4 days refrigerated +	1 day at room temperature =	**50 days**
Proper	40 days frozen +	4 days refrigerated +	1 day at room temperature =	**45 days**

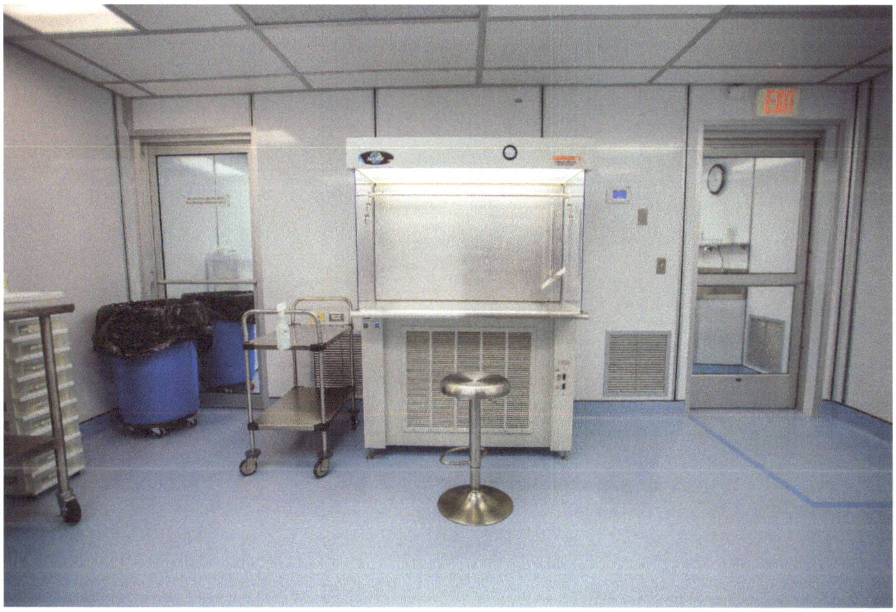

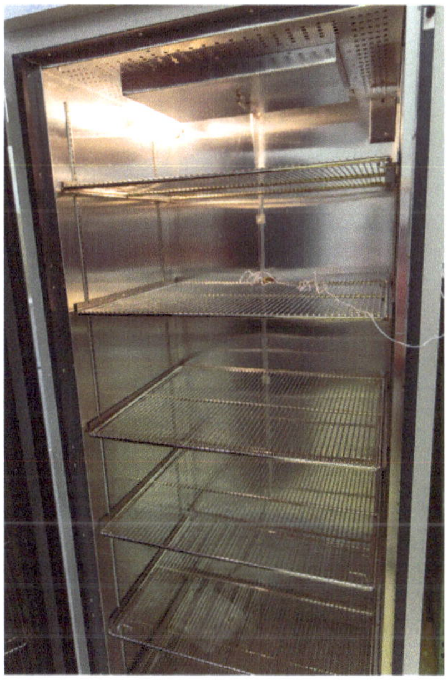

Photos courtesy of Contec, Inc.

total days and exceeds the maximum allowed BUD according to the limits described in Table 2 of USP <797>. Once a CSP has been stored under one condition, the CSP must adhere to the shorter of the BUDs.

Multi-Dose Containers

A CSP compounded as a multi-dose container, one that is intended to be entered or penetrated multiple times and contains a preservative, must be compounded as a Category 2 or 3 CSP. A multi-dose CSP must additionally pass antimicrobial effectiveness testing which is outlined in USP Chapter <51> Antimicrobial Effectiveness. Once this type of CSP is entered or punctured, the multi-dose container must not be used for longer than the assigned BUD or 28 days if supported by antimicrobial effectiveness testing, whichever is shorter.

Summary

BUDs are necessary to help decrease the risk posed to patients receiving sterile, intravenous medications. They provide an alert to health care practitioners, patients, and caregivers to ensure patient safety from sterile preparations by preventing their use when the sterility and quality of the CSP may be compromised. In assigning BUDs, be sure you are considering both the stability of the medication and the sterility risk, as defined by USP <797> in the CSP category tables.

References

1. United States Pharmacopeia. <797> Pharmaceutical Compounding—Sterile Preparations. Revision. November 2022.
2. United States Pharmacopeia. BUD Scientific Rationale for the 2021 Proposed Revisions to <797>. September 1, 2021.

Summary: Categories of Compounded Sterile Preparations (CSPs) and Beyond Use Dating (BUD)

The compounding categories can be confusing. This table provides a general overview comparing Category 1, 2, and 3 CSPs.

	Category 1	Category 2	Category 3
Where is the primary engineering control (PEC) located?	In a segregated compounding area	In an ISO Class 7 buffer room served by an ISO Class 7/8 anteroom	In an ISO Class 7 buffer room served by an ISO Class 7/8 anteroom
Is sterility testing required?	No	Maybe, if longer BUDs are to be assigned	Yes
Is endotoxin testing required?	No	Maybe, if non-sterile ingredients are used and if a BUD is assigned that requires sterility testing. Applies to injectables only.	Yes, if non-sterile ingredients are used. Applies to injectables only.
What BUD can be assigned?	Up to 12 hours room temperature or up to 24 hours refrigerated	Greater than 12 hours room temperature or 24 hours refrigerated	Greater than 12 hours room temperature or 24 hours refrigerated

Category 2 BUDs are more complicated that Category 1 BUDs. This table defines the BUDs that can be assigned for Category 2 CSPs, based on the compounding method and whether sterility testing was performed. This table defines the Category 2 BUDs.[1]

Preparation Details		Storage Conditions		
Compounding method	Sterility testing performed and passed	Controlled room temperature (20 – 25° C or 68 to 77° F)	Refrigerated (2 – 8° C or 36 – 46° F)	Frozen (-25 – -10° C or -13 – 14° F)
Aseptically processed CSPs	No	Prepared from 1 or more non-sterile starting component(s): 1 day	Prepared from 1 or more non-sterile starting component(s): 4 days	Prepared from 1 or more non-sterile starting component(s): 45 days
		Prepared from only sterile starting components: 4 days	Prepared from only sterile starting components: 10 days	Prepared from only sterile starting components: 45 days
	Yes	30 days	45 days	60 days
Terminally sterilized CSPs	No	14 days	28 days	45 days
	Yes	45 days	60 days	90 days

To assign Category 3 BUDs, sterility testing is required, along with other applicable testing. This table defines the Category 3 BUDs.[1]

Preparation and Testing Conditions	Storage Conditions		
	Controlled room temperature (20 – 25° C or 68 – 77° F)	Refrigerated (2 – 8° C or 36 – 46 F)	Frozen (-25 – -10° C or -13 – 14° F)
Aseptically processed CSPs, sterility tested, and passing all applicable tests for Category 3 CSPs	60 days	90 days	120 days
Terminally sterilized CSPs, sterility tested, and passing all applicable tests for Category 3 CSPs	90 days	120 days	180 days

BUD Checklist – When assigning a BUD to a CSP be sure you have evaluated all the following elements:

- ❑ Location of compounding – outside of a PEC, in a PEC in an SCA, or in a PEC in a buffer room
- ❑ Stability of the drug
- ❑ Sterility risks – garbing, material transfer, aseptic technique
- ❑ Starting components – sterile or non-sterile
- ❑ Sterilization technique – filtration or terminal sterilization
- ❑ Final container closure system
- ❑ Storage and transport conditions

If there is still doubt surrounding the appropriate BUD, be conservative. Patient safety must be the number 1 priority.

References

1. United States Pharmacopeia. <797> Pharmaceutical Compounding—Sterile Preparations. Revision. November 2022.

UNIT 3

Facilities and Engineering Controls

This unit will provide an overview of the requirements for meeting the minimum standards described in USP <797> for the structural design of the sterile compounding facility. Ensuring a state of control in all areas where compounding activities are performed is needed to minimize the risk of environmental sources of contamination. A state of control in the compounding facilities is achieved through the use of primary and secondary engineering controls. Primary engineering controls and clean room suites are equipped with high efficiency particulate air (HEPA) filters that capture contaminants (i.e., microbes, dust), thus reducing the risk of airborne contamination. The compounding environment should also be well lit and allow adequate space for the number of employees that will be working simultaneously. A well-designed facility will set home infusion providers up for success and minimize the risk of patient harm from contaminated CSPs.

Primary Engineering Controls (PEC) Examples

- Laminar airflow workbench (LAFW)
- Biological Safety Cabinet (BSC)
- Compounding Aseptic Isolator (CAI)
- Compounding Aseptic Containment Isolator (CACI)
- Integrated Vertical Laminar Flow Zone (IVLFZ)

Secondary Engineering Controls (SEC) Examples

- Clean room suite (anteroom, buffer room)
- Segregated compounding area (SCA)

Secondary Engineering Controls (SECs)

To understand the relationship between primary and secondary engineering controls, we'll first explore secondary engineering controls (SECs) and their functionality. There are 2 types of SECs: clean room suites and segregated compounding areas (SCAs). These compounding areas are very different in both design and functionality. This in turn affects the BUDs that can be assigned to CSPs prepared in these locations. A clean room suite affords the organization the ability to utilize Category 2 and 3 BUDs, which are significantly longer (see Unit 2 Categories of CSPs) and Beyond Use Dating (BUD) for more information). Preparing CSPs in an SCA will limit the BUDs that can be assigned to no more than 12 hours room temperature and 24 hours refrigerated.[1]

Segregated Compounding Areas (SCAs)

Segregated compounding areas (SCAs) are designated spaces or rooms in which a PEC may be placed for

Segregated Compounding Area

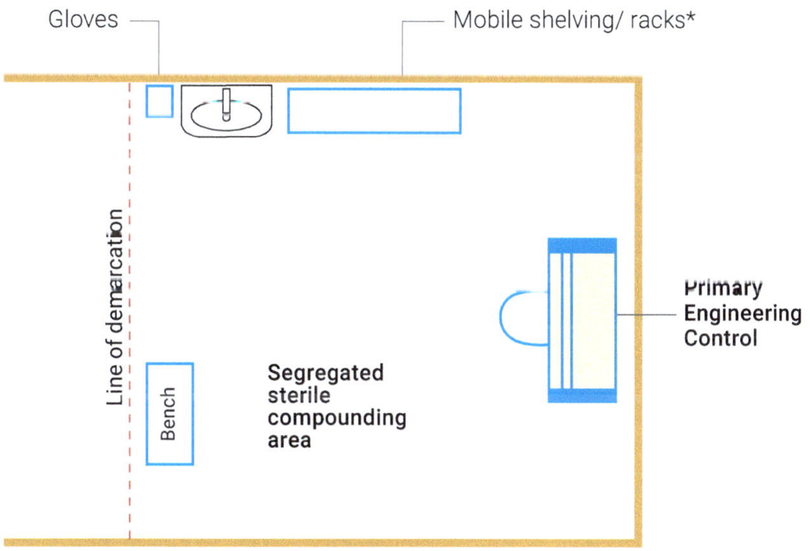

* Other equipment/furniture shown for reference only.

the preparation of non-hazardous medications. The space or area is not ISO Classified, does not have HEPA-filtered air, and does not have any differential pressure requirements. SCAs are not commonly used in home infusion because only Category 1 CSPs can be compounded using this type of facility design and because home infusion pharmacies dispense multiple days' supply at one time, it's not practical. SCAs must not be located near restrooms, traffic areas, warehouse areas, or food preparation areas and must be clearly demarcated.[1]

To identify the area designated as the SCA, there must be a perimeter. This perimeter is a visible demarcation that defines the SCA boundaries, either by a visible line or a wall. In a facility with an SCA design, the sink must be accessible for hand hygiene but located at least 1 meter away from the PEC.

Clean Room Suite

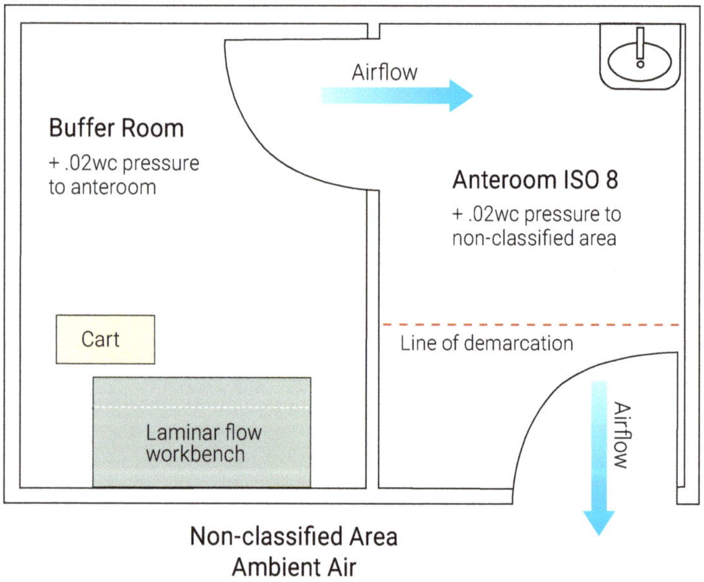

Clean Room Suite

A home infusion facility designed to prepare non-hazardous CSPs must have an anteroom and a buffer room, referred to as the clean room suite. The clean room suite serves as an SEC, protecting CSPs from contamination introduced from the surrounding area. The anteroom and buffer room must have fixed walls and doors and other controls to minimize the flow of lower-quality air into the space.[1] It's important to understand the differences between the buffer room and the anteroom.

Buffer Room: The PEC is located within the buffer room. This room must meet ISO Class 7 air cleanliness requirements. The buffer room must be served by an ISO Class 7 or 8 anteroom. If this design is in place, Category 2 or 3 CSPs can be compounded in this environment.[1]

Anteroom: The anteroom serves as transitional space where hand hygiene, garbing (donning and doffing), staging of components, and other activities occur that have the ability to increase the risk of particulate generation. It is essentially the "buffer area" between the buffer room and the unclassified space. The anteroom must meet ISO Class 8 air cleanliness requirements if it serves a non-hazardous drug buffer room, and it must meet ISO Class 7 if it serves a hazardous drug (HD) buffer room.[1] If a PEC used for sterile compounding is located in the anteroom, it may only be used to prepare Category 1 CSPs because it is essentially the same as a SCA.

Successful clean room suite functionality depends on 3 engineering control design tenets.

1. Airflow and ventilation
2. Segregation
3. Temperature and humidity

Airflow and Ventilation

Standards for Air Quality

USP <797> identifies environmental air quality standards that are consistent with the International Organization for Standardization (ISO) classification for particulate matter in room air found in ISO-14644-1.[2] This classification is achieved through the use of HEPA filters, which must be located in the ceiling of the clean room suite.[1] The level of control of environmental air is determined by the number of airborne particles per cubic meter, which may be influenced by airflow within the PEC, the number of room air changes per hour (ACPH), and air pressure gradients between the various areas within a clean room suite. Exhibit 1 provides the allowable particulates for each ISO Class and which ISO Classes apply to sterile compounding.

Exhibit 1

International Organization of Standardization (ISO) Classification of Particulate Matter in Room Air[1] ISO Class

Class	Allowable Particles / m^3	USP <797> Application
3	35.2	
4	352	
5	3,250	PEC
6	35,200	
7	352,000	Buffer room, HD anteroom
8	3,520,000	Non-HD anteroom

> High-efficiency particulate air (HEPA) filtration is defined as being, using, or containing a filter designed to remove 99.97% of airborne particles measuring 0.3 microns or greater in diameter passing through it.[1]

Air Changes Per Hour

Air in the classified environments must be continuously circulated through the HEPA filters to remove particles. This air movement results in a turbulent flow room, which is different than the unidirectional airflow in a PEC. This constant circulation of air in and out of the room is what is known as air changes per hour (ACPH). There must be enough ACPH, provided by HEPA-filtered airflow, in the clean room suite to maintain the appropriate ISO classification in the buffer and anterooms. Factors that affect the number of required ACPH are:

- Number of personnel required to work in the area
- Number of particulates that may be generated from activities related to compounding
- Equipment (i.e. refrigerators, PECs, and compounding equipment)
- Room pressure
- Temperature

Essentially the more activity in the clean room suite, the more ACPH needed to maintain ISO Classification.

> **You may have heard the phrase *"the solution to pollution is dilution."***
> This is exactly how a turbulent airflow room works. HEPA filtered air mixes with and dilutes airborne contaminants, reducing the concentration within the environment. A turbulent airflow design takes longer to remove contamination than unidirectional airflow. This is because the air turbulence keeps particles suspended and the dilution process is dependent on the volume of air cycling through the space.[3] But this is acceptable, as a unidirectional clean room suite is not a practical application for sterile compounding.

USP <797> requires a minimum of 30 ACPH for ISO Class 7 areas and 20 for ISO Class 8 areas. A higher ACPH may be required to maintain ISO 7 and 8 conditions in facilities needing to mitigate the particulate generation from multiple personnel working simultaneously or from high particulate-generating activities. For ISO Class 7 rooms, at least 15 ACPH must come from the HVAC system while the remainder may come from PECs. If the air provided by PECs is used to meet the necessary ACPH, then those PECs must not be turned off except for during scheduled maintenance. For ISO Class 8 rooms, at least 15 ACPH are required to come from the HVAC system. Exhibit 2 outlines the requirements for ACPH.

Exhibit 2

Summary of ACPH Requirements for Non-Hazardous Drug Compounding[1]

Compounding Area	ACPH Requirement
Unclassified SCA	None
ISO Class 7 Room	30 ACPH At least 15 ACPH from the HVAC system
ISO Class 8 Room	20 ACPH At least 15 ACPH from the HVAC system

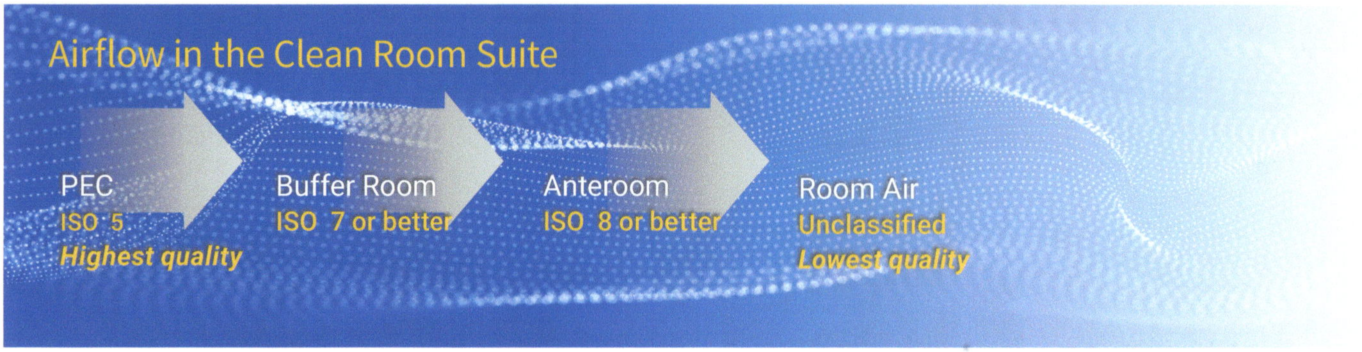

Ventilation

We've just discussed how ACPH are supplied through HEPA filtration. But if we keep adding air to the room, how is it going to exit, taking the particles with it? The air could exit through the room's door, but a more efficient way for the air to exit is through strategically placed low wall returns/exhausts. These returns/exhausts are critical to the functionality of the clean room suite. They pull air from the room, aiding in the maintenance of ISO classification. And having them located low on the wall, creates a general top-down airflow, which prevents particles low on the ground being reintroduced through the room. The number of returns will depend on the size and design of the room. If your returns are not low on the wall, a visual smoke study must be performed to ensure the room can adequately clear particles and there is no stagnant air.[1] This study is discussed in more detail later in this unit.

Segregation

We achieve segregation between the buffer room and anteroom and anteroom and unclassified space through fixed walls and doors, but what happens when the door separating these areas opens? How do we keep dirtier air from flowing into a cleaner area? This segregation is achieved through pressure differential. In a pharmacy preparing non-hazardous Category 2 and 3 CSPs, the environment in the clean room suite must generate a positive pressure in order to sweep air from higher to lower quality. Preventing airflow from unclassified spaces into the clean room is essential for minimizing the potential for airborne contamination. This is accomplished by maintaining a pressure differential between the unclassified room and the anteroom, and between the anteroom and buffer room. A minimum pressure of 0.020-inches water column (inch WC) is required between each ISO area and between the anteroom and unclassified space.[1] See Unit 10 for air pressure requirements for hazardous drug compounding environments.

To ensure the pressure parameters are met, air pressure must be continuously monitored. This may be accomplished through a digital monitor or a magnehelic gauge. In either case, pressure monitoring data must be reviewed and documented at least daily, on days when compounding occurs. The records must be retrievable.[1]

Temperature and Humidity

Temperature and humidity play a critical role in the maintenance of a clean room suite and are controlled through an HVAC system. Ensuring that the HVAC system can manage the heat generated by PECs is crucial and must be considered during planning. It is not possible to add freestanding humidifiers, dehumidifiers, or air conditions to the SEC. The chapter specifies that these devices cannot be in the SEC because of the risk of microbial contamination.

USP <797> suggests that the clean room suite should be maintained at a temperature of 20°C/68°F or cooler and a relative humidity of less than 60%.[1] These parameters decrease the potential for microbial proliferation and provide a comfortable work environment for garbed personnel. Many times a temperature less than 68°F is necessary due to the number of personnel and PECs and other equipment operating in the clean room suite. Although the chapter does not have limits for temperature and humidity, monitoring provides valuable data in the event of a viable sampling excursion.

The temperature and humidity must be recorded each day that compounding occurs either manually or by continuous monitoring devices. All documentation must be stored and retrievable for regulatory inspections and accreditation. USP <797> does indicate that *"the temperature and humidity readings must be reviewed as described in the facility's standard operating procedures (SOPs)."*[1] This leaves it to the organization to decide what a review of the data looks like.

Practical Solution: *Facility managers should set temperature and humidity action limits. Because the chapter supplies only recommended maximum values, but not limits, identify acceptable risk-based limits for the individual facility. Inspectors and surveyors will expect to see a plan in place in the event the recommended levels are exceeded. If limits are set and documented in SOPs, it's not necessary to follow USP's recommendation. Just be sure to capture the rationale for the chosen limits.*

Today, many organizations use digital temperature and humidity sensors that are connected to a building management system that continuously monitors and alerts designated pharmacy personnel when action limits are exceeded.

Design Elements and Finishes

Facility design must be based on workflow. Movement (e.g., personnel activity, transfer of materials) within the clean room suite or SCA and PECs can disrupt the functioning of the engineering controls by creating airflow disturbances. Workflow should also be designed to limit the introduction of contaminants into the ISO-certified areas or SCA where compounding is taking place. Whether you are designing a new space or reevaluating your current sterile compounding space, be sure that only the furniture, equipment, and essential materials for performing compounding processes are permitted in the clean room suite or SCA. Also consider future needs in your design, such space for additional PECs and power and data outlets.

The appropriate finishes are essential to the success of the clean room suite. Improper finishes can contribute to high particle counts, microbial excursions, and insanitary conditions, such as rust.[4] USP <797> requires that all surfaces in the clean room suite be smooth, nonporous, non-shedding, and free from cracks and crevices.[1] Think about your current clean room suite. Do the surfaces meet this chapter requirement? If not, what changes could be made to be compliant? The chapter also indicates that the surfaces ***should*** be resistant to damage by cleaning agents.[1] Ultimately, you want the surfaces to be able to withstand frequent cleaning.

Because the chapter requires surfaces to be free from cracks and crevices, it only makes sense that any junctures between walls, floors, and ceilings must be sealed to prevent the accumulation of dust and dirt. Any penetrations through the ceiling or walls must be sealed.[1]

Practical Solution: *Use a silicone sealant to fill any junctures in the clean room suite. Silicone will break down overtime, so it is important to regularly check the condition of the silicone and replace as needed. The best time to check for the integrity is during the monthly clean. Those who do the monthly clean should be trained to report issues to the designated person.*

Classified areas should minimize dust-collecting overhangs, such as utility pipes, ledges, and windowsills. If overhangs or ledges are present, they must be easily cleanable.[1] These types of designs may be seen in older sterile compounding clean rooms. Although overhangs and ledges are acceptable, with proper cleaning, new clean room designs are moving away from these elements.

The anteroom must have a line of demarcation (LOD) that separates the clean and dirty side of the anteroom. The dirty side of the room opens into the unclassified space, and the clean side is closest to the buffer room. The LOD must be a visible line.[1] This is best accomplished by heat welding a line into the sheet vinyl floor or using different floor colors for the clean side and dirty side.

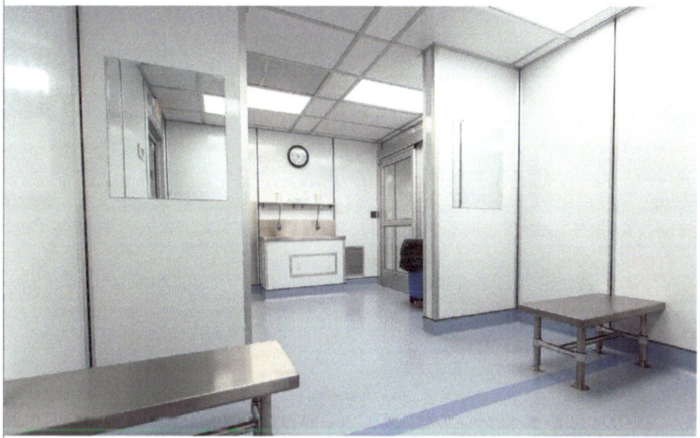

Photo courtesy of Contec, Inc.

Practical Solution: *If your facility does not have a visible LOD, clean room grade tape can be used to create a line. Be sure to check the integrity of the tape regularly, as defined in your SOP, and replace the tape when it starts to peel or flake.*

USP <797> addresses water sources in the clean room suite, as it can be a significant risk of microbial contamination. Sinks are allowed in the anteroom to accommodate hand hygiene; however, an organization may choose to have its sink outside of the anteroom. The buffer room must not contain plumbed water sources, such as eyewashes and the clean room suite

Exhibit 3
Design Element Chapter Specifications and Practical Solutions

Design Element	Chapter <797> [1]	Practical Solution

Door	• Door seals and sweeps **should not** be installed between buffer and anterooms
	• Doors **should** be hands-free
		• Interlocking doors to limit buffer room and anteroom doors opening at the same time
		• Door opening wide enough to support the movement of personnel, equipment, and product
		• Recommended materials[5]
		  ○ Anodized aluminum
		  ○ 2-component epoxy painted hollow metal
		  ○ Hygienic fiberglass reinforced polymer (FRP) with a smooth surface texture without wood core

Wall	• **Must be** constructed of, or may be covered with, durable material and the integrity of the surface must be maintained • Panels **must** be joined together and sealed to each other and the support structure	• Apply 2-component epoxy paint to all exposed gypsum wall board • Cover wall with a smooth, heavy-gauge polymer wall panel[5]

Ceiling	• Inlaid panels **must** be caulked around each panel to seal them to the support frame	• Unfinished gypsum wall board[5]
		  ○ Apply 2-component epoxy paint to all exposed gypsum wall board
		  ○ Cover with a smooth heavy-gauge polymer wall panel
		• Inlaid ceiling panels[5]
		  ○ Smooth texture
		  ○ Non-perforated
		  ○ Square lay-in
		  ○ Clean room-rated panels

Floor	• **Must** include coving to the sidewall, or
	• The juncture between the floor and the wall **must** be caulked
		• Smooth and sealed with continuous, welded seams (no tiles)[5]
		  ○ Resilient homogenous type sheet vinyl or rubber products recommended for use in hygienic/clean room areas
		  ○ Epoxy laid flooring that is smooth, but slip resistant

Pass-through chambers, including cart pass-throughs	• Both doors **must** never be opened at the same time • Doors **should** be interlocking	• Interlocking doors • Made from stainless steel and glass • Seamless internal chamber • Gasketed doors • Sturdy, cleanable hinges
Ceiling light fixtures	Exterior lens surface **must** be smooth, mounted flush, and sealed	Clean room grade
Shelving and carts	**Must** be constructed from nonporous materials with cleanable casters and wheels	• Stainless steel, solid surface, or hard plastic • Casters for ease of cleaning • Solid, flat shelves (not wire)
Sink	**Should** enable hands-free use	• Stainless steel • Hands-free • No strainer • Deep enough to wash to the elbows
Furniture and equipment	• Only items necessary for compounding activities are permitted • **Should** be low-shedding and easily cleaned • Number, design, location, and manner of installation **must not** impact air quality	• Place equipment, like refrigerators*, by returns/exhausts • Clean room grade, when possible **Compressorless refrigerators help minimize particle generation*

must not contain floor drain(s). Another potential water source is the sprinkler system, which is likely to be required due to life safety codes. If a sprinkler system is installed, it should be recessed and covered, and the covers should be easily cleanable.[1]

It can be challenging to identify the chapter design requirements and determine what is appropriate for your clean room suite. Exhibit 3 (see opposite page) breaks down various design elements into chapter requirements and industry accepted practical solutions.

Pass-Through Chamber

Pass-through chambers are a valuable design feature. They offer convenience in material transfer and limit unnecessary entry into the classified environment. Those who are designing a new clean room suite often have a lot of questions as to where to place these pass-through chambers and what type of pass-through chamber to install. To complicate things, regulatory documents do not have the same requirements. Let's look at what is required when it comes to pass-through chambers.

USP <797> does not require pass-through chambers to interlock and does not require HEPA filtration.[1] However, FDA's Insanitary Conditions document states that *"material flow directly between an unclassified area and a room in which sterile compounding is conducted (e.g., unclassified pass-through chambers)"* is considered an insanitary condition. Having an unclassified pass-through chamber between an unclassified space and a buffer room is a common, efficient design, allowed by USP <797>. This begs the question, which is the right design choice? What you decide will likely be based on your risk tolerance and your state regulations.

There are some things to consider when deciding on pass-through chamber location and design:[6]

1. The FDA expects HEPA-filtered pass-through chambers between classified and unclassified areas, even though this is not required by the chapter.
2. HEPA-filtered pass-through chambers are more expensive than a pass-through without HEPA-filtration.
3. HEPA-filtered pass-through chambers are much larger and need electrical connections. Depending on your existing design it may not be possible to install a HEPA-filtered pass-through chambers due to space constraints and availability of electricity.
4. Certification of HEPA-filtered pass-through chambers is required every 6 months.
5. Pass-through chambers, whether HEPA-filtered or not, are best installed between the unclassified space and the buffer room. This provides the most efficient workflow and reduces personnel traffic in the anteroom. This is especially important in an ISO Class 7 anteroom, which may struggle to maintain acceptable viable air levels.

SCA Finishes

The requirements for finishes in the SCA are very different from the requirements for a clean room suite. All surfaces in the SCA:[1]

1. **Must** be clean, uncluttered, and dedicated to compounding
2. **Should** be smooth, impervious, free from cracks and crevices, and non-shedding
3. **Should** be resistant to damage by cleaning agents, sporicidal and other types of disinfectants, and tools used to clean

Exhibit 4
SCA and Clean Room Suite Summary Comparison

SCA	Clean Room Suite
Unclassified	ISO classified
HEPA-filtration not required	HEPA-filtration
ACPH not required	Specific ACPH requirements
No pressure requirements*	Pressure requirements
Comfortable work conditions	Monitored temperature and humidity
Perimeter line	Line of demarcation

* Containment segregated compounding areas (C-SCAs) do have pressure requirements. C-SCAs are discussed in Unit 10.

As with the clean room suite, dust-collecting overhangs and ledges should be minimized. And if they are present, they must be easily cleanable.[1]

Practical Solution: *Outfitting the SCA with the same finishes used in a clean room suite will help ensure the longevity of the surfaces and their ability to withstand repeated cleaning with bactericidal and sporicidal cleaning and disinfecting agents.*

Primary Engineering Controls (PECs)

Compared to secondary engineering controls, primary engineering controls are simple devices, that provide ISO Class 5 air cleanliness for sterile compounding. It's important to understand how PECs function, so

Exhibit 5:
Categories of LAFS and the Types of PECs That Belong to Each

- **Laminar Airflow System (LAFS)**
  - Laminar Airflow Workbench (LAFW)
  - Integrated Vertical Laminar Airflow Zones (IVLFZ)
  - Class II Biological Safety Cabinet (BSC)
- **Restricted-Access Barrier System (RABS)**
  - Compounding Aseptic Isolator (CAI)
  - Compounding Aseptic Containment Isolator (CACI)
- **Isolator**

they can be properly used for the preparation of sterile medications. Although there are many different PECs available for sterile compounding, there are some USP <797> requirements regarding the functionality and placement of PECs that apply to all these devices. The PEC must:[1]

1. Provide unidirectional airflow
2. Supply HEPA-filtered air at a velocity capable of sweeping particles away from critical sites
3. Be placed in a way to accommodate cleaning the area around and under them

Unidirectional Airflow

Air within a PEC moving in a single direction in a uniform manner and at sufficient velocity to sweep particles away from the DCA.[1]

Do your PECs meet all these chapter requirements? How do you know?

There are 3 categories of PECs, which include laminar airflow systems (LAFS), restricted-access barrier systems (RABS), and pharmaceutical isolators. The category of LAFS can be further broken down into 3 types of PECs, which include laminar airflow workbenches (LAFWs), integrated vertical laminar airflow zones (IVLFZs), and Class II biological safety cabinets (BSCs). The category of RABS consists of 2 types of PECs, a compounding aseptic isolator (CAI) and compounding aseptic containment isolator (CACI). All of these ISO Class 5 devices have very specific characteristics that make them unique. Exhibit 5 provides a visual representation of the categories and the devices that belong to each.

Do you know which PECs are used in your sterile compounding operation? Do you know why each device was chosen?

Airflow Direction

PECs are available in 2 different airflow directions: horizontal and vertical.

In horizontal airflow, the HEPA filter is in the back of the device and air moves from the back of the device toward the front of the device.

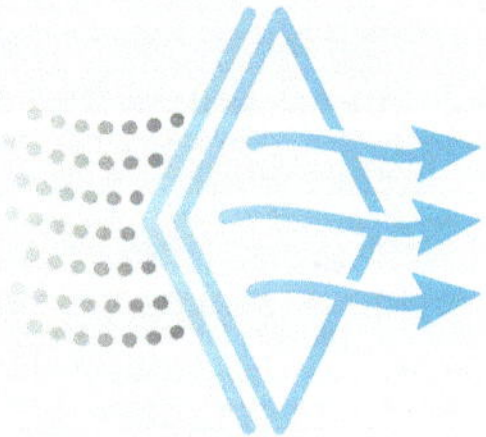

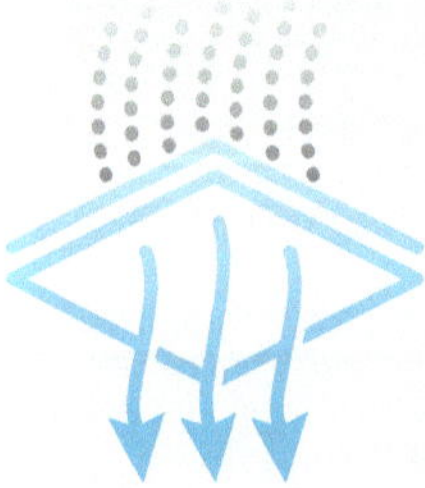

In vertical airflow, the HEPA filter is in the top of the device and air moves from the top of the device towards the work surface of the device.

Which airflow do you work in?

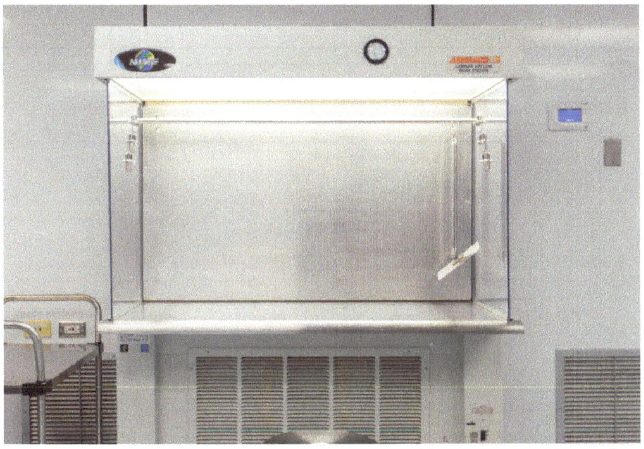

Horizontal LAFW — Photo courtesy of Contec, Inc.

Laminar Airflow Systems

LAFS are designed to provide unidirectional, HEPA-filtered airflow to protect the direct compounding area (DCA). These ISO Class 5 devices are all slightly different in design and the airflow direction provided. Let's explore the different types of LAFS.

Laminar Airflow Workbenches (LAFWs)

LAFWs are the most commonly used PEC for the preparation of non-hazardous sterile medications. These devices provide ISO Class 5 air or better through either horizontal or vertical unidirectional HEPA-filtered airflow. LAFWs only provide protection to the preparations and do not afford protection to personnel using the device. Therefore, these devices are not appropriate for the preparation of hazardous CSPs or for weighing and measuring active pharmaceutical ingredient (API)

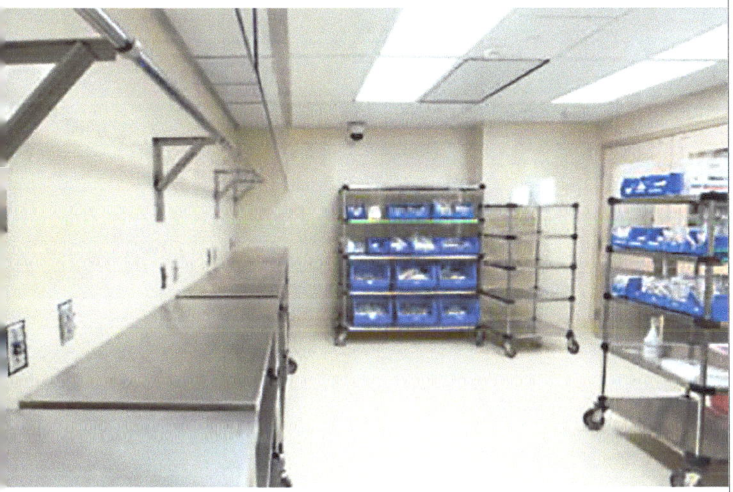

Photo courtesy of Contec, Inc.

> The use of vertical LAFWs and IVLFZs (as seen above) is becoming more common for facilities that use automated compounding devices for parenteral nutrition (PN).

Integrated Vertical Laminar Flow Zones (IVLFZs)

An IVLFZ is a designated area serving as the PEC within an ISO Class 7 or cleaner buffer room. Essentially, the PEC is built into the buffer room and as the name suggests, it provides vertical airflow. IVLFZs cannot be placed in SCAs.

IVLFZs are created by placing HEPA filters over the entire worksurface and effective placement of air returns. In addition, the unidirectional HEPA-filtered zone must be separated from the buffer room with a physical barrier. This barrier is used to direct the HEPA-filtered air downward over the work area to separate the DCA from the rest of the buffer room.

IVLFZs can be beneficial in sterile compounding operations where large, automated compounding devices, such as compounders for PN, are utilized. However, this type of design comes with challenges. Dynamic airflow smoke pattern tests have shown it very difficult to meet the requirements and design to achieve unidirectional airflow under dynamic operating conditions.[1] As with LAFWs, IVLFZs are not appropriate for preparation of hazardous CSPs or for weighing and measuring API.

> **What are dynamic operating conditions?**
> USP <797> defines dynamic operating conditions as *"conditions in the compounding area in which operating personnel are present and simulating or performing compounding. The conditions should reflect the largest number of personnel and highest complexity of compounding expected during routine operations as determined by the designated person(s)."*[1]

Class II Biological Safety Cabinets

Class II BSCs are ventilated with an open front and inward and downward (vertical) unidirectional HEPA-filtered airflow and HEPA-filtered exhaust.[1] These devices protect personnel from airborne drugs and provide an ISO Class 5 or better environment. Although BSCs could be used for non-hazardous compounding, they are most commonly used for the preparation of HDs. There are 3 different types of Class II BSCs that can be used for HD preparation, Type A2, Type B2, and Type C1. BSCs will be covered in more detail in Unit 10 of this module, which discusses HD compounding.

Placement of LAFS

There are 2 things to consider as part of LAFS placement. First, is BUD assignment. The LAFS must be in an ISO Class 7 or better buffer room for preparing Category 2 and 3 CSPs. Second, is how the placement of the LAFS in the room will affect the functionality of the device. It is critical to locate the LAFS out of high-traffic areas and away from areas in which air currents could disrupt the function of the PEC.

Practical Solution: *High traffic areas, ceiling HEPA filters, and room airflow in the clean room or SCA could result in room air being drawn into the LAFS. As part of certification, your certifier is required to perform smoke studies that will aid in the identification of PEC placement issues. Look for both dynamic and static smoke pattern test results on your report. If you are unsure whether the testing was done or of the results, be sure to talk with your certifier.*

Restricted Access Barrier Systems (RABS)

RABS are enclosed workspaces that provide vertical flow, HEPA-filtered ISO Class 5 unidirectional air. These devices are different from LAFS because they are designed with defined openings that are validated to prevent the transfer of air contamination. RABS have 2 chambers: The main chamber, where sterile compounding occurs and the transfer chamber, which is used to move materials from outside of the RABS to inside the RABS without introducing contamination. RABS also have glove ports that provide separation between the surrounding areas and aseptic processes. As was mentioned, there are 2 types of RABS: a compounding aseptic isolator (CAI) and compounding aseptic containment isolator (CACI). Although both devices have the word isolator in their names, these are not true isolators.

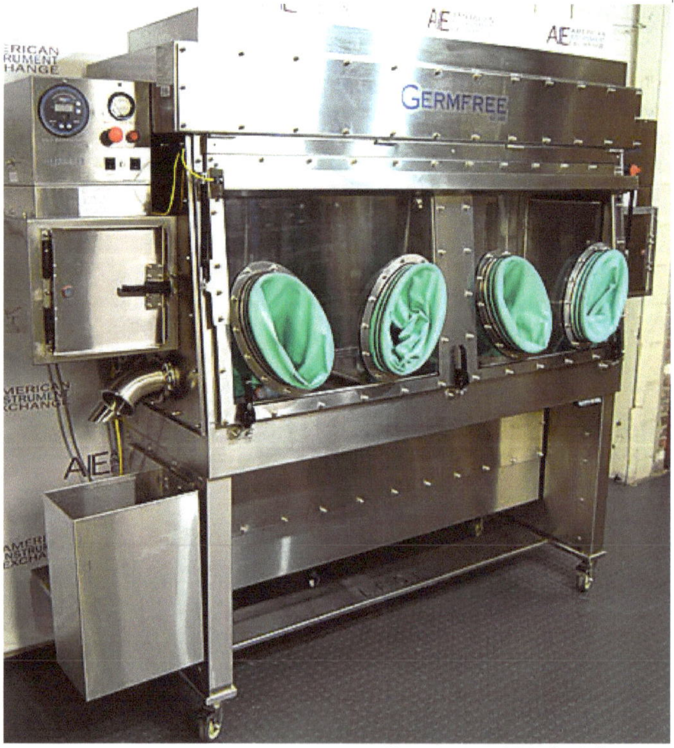

Photo courtesy of Germfree Laboratories

> Although CAIs and CACIs have the word isolator in their names, these are not true isolators and are considered RABS.

Compounding Aseptic Isolator

The CAI is designed to maintain an ISO Class 5 environment throughout the compounding and material transfer processes. It does this through a positive pressure differential, meaning air from the main chamber cascades to the transfer chamber when the door between the 2 chambers is opened and air in the transfer chamber cascades outside the device when the outer transfer chamber door is opened. Because of this positive pressure, the CAI is only suitable for non-hazardous drug compounding.

Compounding Aseptic Containment Isolator

The goal of the CACI design is slightly different than that of the CAI. It is designed to protect the worker from exposure to drugs and provide an ISO Class 5 environment. Because this device provides containment, it is appropriate for hazardous drug preparation. Containment is achieved through a negative pressure differential, meaning that the device is negative to the area around it, and it will draw outside air in. It is critical that the certifer verify the functionality of the device to avoid ingress of unwanted contamination.

Practical Solution: *Check the integrity of the RABS sleeves and change the RABS gloves daily. Holes and tears, especially on CACI sleeves and gloves, will allow for the entry of contamination, posing a safety risk to patients.*

Placement of RABS

As with LAFS, placement of RABS depends on the desired BUD. If preparing Category 1 compounds, the RABS can be placed in unclassified air in an SCA;

however, if it is used to compound Category 2 or 3 CSPs, the RABS must be placed in a clean room suite with ISO Class 7 or better buffer room and ISO Class 8 anteroom.[1]

Pharmaceutical Isolators

Pharmaceutical isolators provide protection from the surrounding area to maintain ISO Class 5 air quality during dynamic conditions. However, they are very different from the other devices already discussed. There are 4 components of an isolator[1]:

1. Controlled workspace
2. Transfer device(s)
3. Access device(s)
4. Integral decontamination system

If you are not familiar with pharmaceutical isolators, you will notice that the first 3 components are like a RABS. What makes this device so different is the integrated decontamination system. Overall, a well-designed pharmaceutical isolator offers a significant increase in sterility assurance, but the use, care, and maintenance are very different than that of traditional sterile compounding PECs.[7] Maintenance and qualification and requalification of the decontamination cycle would be done by a vendor. Also, the faster decontamination cycles take 1 hour, many take longer.[8] Because of this, pharmaceutical isolators are not typically used in sterile compounding.

Placement of Pharmaceutical Isolators

Isolator placement is a bit different than that of other PECs. Placing the isolator in an SCA still only allows for Category 1 compounding. However, those compounding Category 2 and 3 CSPs can place the isolator in an ISO Class 8 positive pressure room and are not required to have the traditional buffer room/anteroom clean room suite. Isolators can be used for hazardous drug compounding per USP <800> standards.[1]

Exhibit 6 provides a comparison of the different PECs discussed in this Unit. You will notice that there is no benefit to choosing a particular device because they all afford the same BUD options for Category 2 and 3 CSPs. With all these options, you want to consider the following when choosing the best PEC for your location:

1. Airflow direction – Aseptic technique in horizontal flow comes more naturally than when working in vertical flow.
2. Type of compounding – Working with HDs will limit you to containment PECs.
3. Ease of use – LAFWs and BSCs are easier to work in than RABS, resulting in better compliance to SOPs.

Certification

You've likely been present during a PEC or clean room certification. Have you ever thought about what the certifier is testing when they come to your facility or why what they do is important?

Certification, which is a series of tests, ensures the engineering controls are meeting specific parameters. The primary engineering controls and clean room suite in your facility are worthless if they do not meet design and air quality specifications, making certification an essential part of ensuring patient safety. Certification of the classified areas

Exhibit 6
PEC Comparison

PEC	Airflow	Use	Location	
			Category 1	Category 2 or 3
LAFW	Horizontal or Vertical	Non-hazardous	SCA	ISO Class and buffer room with ISO Class 7 or 8 anteroom
IVLFZ	Vertical	Non-hazardous	N/A	
CAI	Vertical	Non-hazardous	SCA	
BSC	Vertical	Non-hazardous or hazardous	SCA	
CACI	Vertical	Hazardous	SCA	
Isolator	Vertical	Non-hazardous or hazardous	SCA	ISO Class 8 positive pressure room

Certification is an essential part of ensuring patient safety.

must be performed initially, before the use of the engineering control, and every 6 months thereafter. USP <797> provides guidance on the testing required but does not indicate that engineering control be tested to any specific standards or guidance. It is recommended that sterile compounding engineering controls be certified according to Controlled Environment Testing Association (CETA) Application Guide (CAG)-003, titled Certification of Sterile Compounding Facilities for USP Compliance.

CAG-003 is an all-encompassing testing guide that combines the testing requirements from various industry standards and guidelines. Check your certification report. If it indicates the certifier tested to CAG-003, the facility is complying with the chapter. If not, you will likely see a variety of testing standards listed, which should match those listed as references in CAG-003. If you are still not sure as to how your engineering controls were tested, get clarification from the certification company and ask for clearer documentation on the testing report.

There is one other important note regarding certification testing and the standards and guidelines that are to be followed for the testing. USP <797> does not list all the required PEC-specific tests, however CAG-003 does.

What is CETA? Controlled Environment Testing Association (CETA) is a non-profit organization dedicated to promoting and developing quality assurance within the controlled environment testing industry.[9] It has developed several CETA Application Guides (CAGs) that outline the testing needs of sterile compounding facilities. In addition, it has created a testing exam and credential for those who service sterile compounding facilities, called the Registered Certification Professional – Sterile Compounding Facilities (RCP-SCF).

Exhibit 7
Required Clean Room Testing

Clean Room Suite	PEC
Airflow testing	Airflow testing
HEPA filter integrity testing	HEPA filter integrity testing
Total particle count testing	Total particle count testing
Room segregation (pressure differential)	Dynamic airflow smoke pattern test
Visual smoke study*	PEC-specific tests**
Temperature and humidity*	

* The visual smoke study is only required if the returns/exhausts are not located low on the wall. Temperature and humidity are optional tests but are commonly performed by many certifiers.

** These tests are defined in CAG-002 Compounding Isolator Testing Guide and CAG-003.

Practical Solution: *Certification responsibilities are shared by both the certification company and the sterile compounding organization. Consider having a quality agreement in place with the certification company. This document clearly identifies the responsibilities of each party and sets service expectations. As part of the quality agreement, be sure to request training records of the certification technician onsite at your location and SOPs describing their testing and reporting procedures.*

You also should provide the certifier with your SOPs before they arrive, so they know what to expect when garbing and transferring their test equipment.

USP <797> lists 4 tests that are part of certification.

1. Airflow testing
2. HEPA filter integrity testing
3. Total particle count testing
4. Dynamic airflow smoke pattern test

This simplistic listing in the chapter is actually very complicated. Let's breakdown this testing into what is required for clean room suites and PECs.

Organizations can request that the certifiers at your facility hold a CETA credential or at least have an on-site lead who is CETA credentialed.

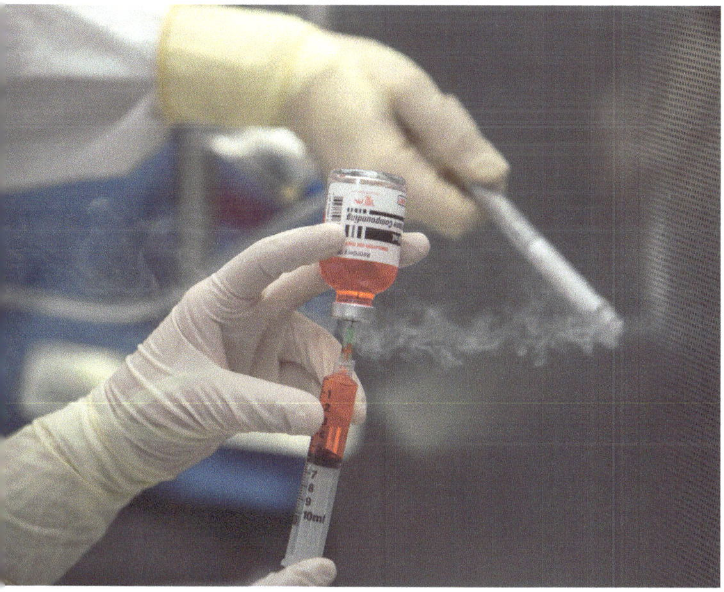

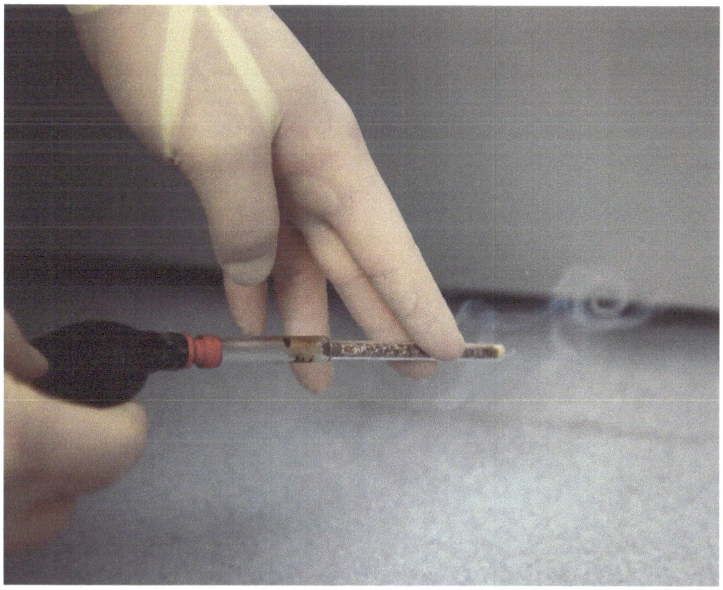

Photos courtesy of Contec, Inc.

Airflow Testing

Airflow testing in both the PEC and clean room are performed to ensure the HEPA-filtered airflow is adequate to maintain the desired ISO classification. For the clean room suite, the total airflow from the HEPA filters and the PECs is used to calculate the air changes per hour for each room. When testing the airflow in the PEC, multiple velocity readings of the air leaving the HEPA filter are recorded. These readings are used to verify that the airflow velocity is uniform and appropriate to the specific PEC, as per manufacturers' specifications.

HEPA Filter Integrity Testing

The integrity of the HEPA filter is essential, as filters with significant leaks can allow contamination to enter the ISO classified space. HEPA filter integrity testing verifies that the filters are free from leaks greater than the allowed percentage. Notice it says greater than the allowable percentage. No filter is totally leak free, but you may see "zero leakage" on your report. If it is reported this way, it means the filter leakage is acceptable.

This testing is done on the filter before it leaves the manufacturer and must be done when the filter is installed and at every certification. This not only includes the filters in the PECs and ceiling but also those in HEPA-filtered pass-through chambers. This is one of the more challenging clean room tests for certifiers to complete because they need to introduce an aerosol challenge upstream of the filter. If there is no way to do this, the test cannot be performed, resulting in non-compliance. Be sure your certifier has a mechanism to leak test the filter. In the event there is a leak, the certifier may be able to repair it, if it is does not block or restrict airflow more than 3% of the entire filter face area and no single repair has a lesser (width) dimension exceeding 1.5" (3.8cm).[10,11] Otherwise, the filter will need to be replaced.

Total Particle Count Testing

Total particle count testing is used to determine the ISO Class air cleanliness of an area under dynamic conditions. This testing is performed using a calibrated particle counter and measures particles 0.5 microns and larger in size. The number of sample locations is based on the area of the space sampled. ISO-14644-1 provides a table that is used to determine the number of locations.[2]

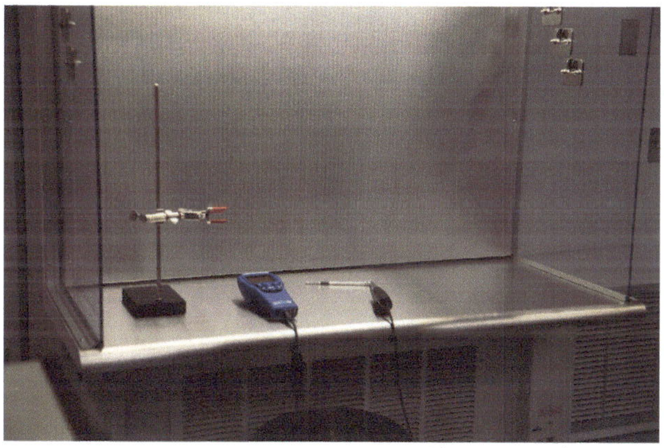

Photo courtesy of Contec, Inc.

Room Segregation

Room segregation, also known as pressure differential, is not specifically listed as a test in USP <797>, but it is mentioned as part of the airflow testing. Room pressure differential in doorways between adjacent rooms is necessary to ensure consistent airflow from an area of higher air quality to an area of equal or lower air quality. For example, an ISO Class 7 buffer room flows into a dirtier ISO Class 8 anteroom, indicating positive pressure, while an ISO Class 7 anteroom flows into an equally classified HD buffer room, indicating negative pressure. The certifier will measure the pressure readings from each door to the adjacent space. They may also verify the airflow direction with a smoke source.

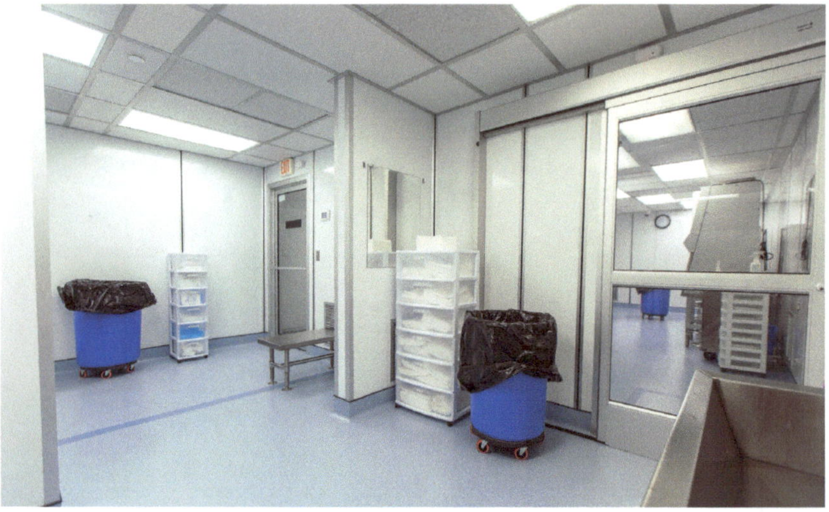

Photo courtesy of Contec, Inc.

> All testing should be conducted under dynamic conditions, including the number of personnel typically in the room performing normal daily operations. Ensure that the certifier documents the number of people in the room at the time of testing in their report.

Visual Smoke Study

The clean room suite will need a visual smoke study if the returns/exhausts are not located low on the wall.[1] This is because air in the clean room suite is turbulent and if the clean room is not designed with ceiling HEPAs and low wall returns/exhausts, dirty air from the floor will be pulled up towards the ceiling. This design could also result in stagnant air. In the visual smoke study, a visible source of smoke, which is neutrally buoyant, is used to verify an absence of stagnant airflow where particulates can accumulate. This study does not need to be performed under dynamic operating conditions.[1]

Temperature and Humidity

Temperature and humidity testing are not required USP <797> certification tests, but many certifiers will provide this data in their clean room test reports. It is simply a snapshot in time of the conditions during certification. If viable air and surface samples are conducted in conjunction with certification, the data can also provide insight into the cause of any possible excursions.

Dynamic Airflow Smoke Pattern Test

The dynamic airflow smoke pattern test is performed in every PEC *"during dynamic operating conditions to demonstrate unidirectional airflow and sweeping action over and away from the preparation(s)."*[1] A visible source of smoke, which is neutrally buoyant, is used to observe air patterns in the PEC and identify the DCA. This testing is done with surrogate materials, simulating compounding manipulations. The simulation must be done by 1 of your staff members, so be sure someone is available to assist in the testing.

The reporting of this test should include a statement detailing the airflow patterns and whether it was acceptable, in addition to clear identification of the DCA.

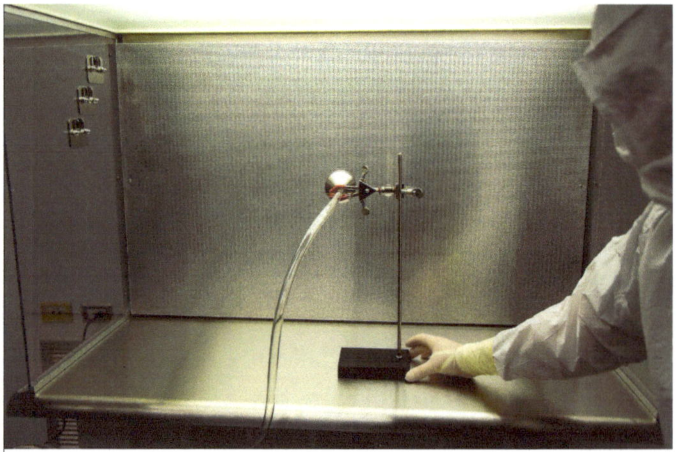

Photo courtesy of Contec, Inc.

Dynamic Airflow Smoke Pattern Testing as a Training Tool – Yes, dynamic airflow smoke pattern testing is a required certification test, but it can also be used an exceptional training tool. A few suggestions for incorporate this into training.

1. Share the videos captured during certification with staff.
2. Rotate staff who assist during the testing.
3. Invest in smoke equipment and use it during the training of staff.

Understanding PEC airflow is an essential part of good aseptic technique. Having a visual of the air flow patterns in the PEC will give staff a new appreciation of first air and aid in technique improvement.

> You can search for accredited BSC certification professionals on NSF's website: nsf.org/

The best way to document this testing is through a video recording in conjunction with a written description.

Practical Solution: *In addition to performing the required dynamic airflow smoke pattern testing, static testing is a useful tool for identifying proper placement of compounding equipment, such as automated compounding devices (ACDs) and workflow management systems. Excessive refluxing of air and the inability for the air to effectively exit the PEC may require raising the equipment off the work surface to allow for better air flow.*

PEC-Specific Tests

Depending on the type of PEC, there is additional testing that must be performed in the device to verify functionality. Review certification reports to be sure this additional testing is completed by the certification company.

LAFWs – In addition to the testing required by USP <797>, CAG-003 indicates LAFWs should also have the induction leak/backstreaming test. *"This test verifies the LAFW is free from unsealed construction joints and that room airflow patterns or bench location do not introduce particulate contamination into the critical work area."*[11] The testing methods are described in CAG-003.

BSCs – Class II BSCs are tested according to NSF/ANSI 49 and should only be tested by certification professionals, who are accredited by NSF International for the certification of Class II BSCs.[11] Three tests are done in addition to the USP <797> required testing. The inflow velocity test measures the manufacturer's design for airflow containment and exhaust. The airflow containment test is made up of 4 separate tests: downflow test, view screen retention test, work opening edge retention test, and sash/window seal test.[12] The site installation assessment verifies the BSC is properly integrated and can notify the user of containment loss, through audible and visual alarms.[12]

RABS – CAIs and CACIs are testing according to CAG-002 Compounding Isolator Testing Guide. Within this CAG, 3 tests, in addition to the USP <797>-required tests, are described. These tests include the chamber pressure test and the ingress and egress test for both CAIs and CACIs, and the particle containment test for CACIs.[13] All of these tests are designed to ensure the integrity and cleanliness of the RABS. In addition, the site installation test that is required for a BSC is also required for a CACI.

Recertification

Although certification is required every 6 months, there are some reasons why testing may need to be performed sooner. These include:[1]

1. Redesign of the facility
2. Construction
   Replacement or relocation of any PEC (Moving a PEC for cleaning the floors and walls under and around the equipment is not considered relocation)
3. Alteration in the configuration of the room that could affect airflow or air quality (If you are not sure if a change will affect the airflow or air quality contact your certifier.)

If you are not sure if certification is needed, contact the certification company and state board of pharmacy for guidance. Consider adding these reasons for certification to your SOPs.

Documentation and Certification Failures

Certification documentation and retention is essential. At the completion of clean room and PEC testing the certifier must provide a comprehensive report. The report and any other certification-associated records must be reviewed by the designated person(s) to ensure that the classified environments are appropriate for use and meet chapter requirements.[1] Some certification companies may leave an interim report until the final report can be prepared. Ask your certification provider is this is an option. Once you receive the final report, it is imperative to conduct a thorough review of all pass and fail findings. Failures will result in immediate action. Reviewing passing results can identify trends that could potentially lead to failure in the future, allowing organizations to be proactive in their environmental monitoring program.

USP <797> does have specific reporting requirements for some testing. As part of airflow testing, the ACPH from HVAC, ACPH contributed from the PEC, and the total ACPH must be documented on the certification report for ISO Class 7 rooms and the total ACPH must be documented on the certification report for ISO Class 8 rooms. The number of personnel present in each PEC and SEC during total particle-count tests and dynamic airflow smoke-pattern tests must be documented on the report. Be sure to check reports for this information.

In the event of any certification failure, the designated person must initiate a corrective action plan. The corrective action plan and the outcome of the corrective actions must be documented. Data collected in response to corrective actions must be reviewed to confirm that the actions taken have been effective.

Practical Solution: *Some certification failures are simple to resolve. If a HEPA filter has a leak, it is repaired or replaced. But some failures may be more complex, such as a room airflow issue. The certification company can be used as a resource in the event of a certification failure. Knowledgeable individuals with the company can assist in resolution and compliance.*

Summary

Primary and secondary engineering controls are essential to patient safety and the success of a sterile compounding organization. At first glance, PEC and SEC functionality appear simple and straightforward, but there are many nuances that go into creating an appropriate environment for the preparation of sterile medications. Understanding the functionality of PECs and SECs, and the testing required to verify that functionality has a positive impact on the workflow and design of an operation.

References

1. United States Pharmacopeial Convention, Inc. General Chapter <797> Pharmaceutical Compounding – Sterile Preparations. November 2022.
2. International Organization for Standardization. ISO 14644-1. Clean rooms And Associated Controlled Environments – Part 1: Classification of Air Cleanliness By Particle Concentration. 2015.
3. Controlled Environment Testing Association. CAG-002-2005. CETA Applications Guide for the use of Compounding Aseptic Isolators in Compounding Sterile Preparations in Healthcare facilities. December 8, 2008.
4. Food and Drug Administration. Insanitary Conditions at Compounding Facilities Guidance for Industry. November 2020.
5. CriticalPoint, LLC. Pearls of Knowledge. Clean room Suite and Segregated Compounding Area Fit and Finishes. March 2019.
6. CriticalPoint, LLC. Pearls of Knowledge. Considerations on the Design and Placement of Pass-throughs for Sterile Compounding. Originally published in March 2017; revised and republished July 2019.
7. Markarian, Jennifer. Pharmaceutical Technology. Best Practices in Using Isolator Technology. Volume 44, Issue 2. February 2, 2020.
8. Denk, Richard. ISPE – PDA Conference Australia Melbourne. Decontamination with H2O2 for Aseptic Isolators. September 20, 2019.
9. Controlled Environment Testing Association. About CETA. cetaintrnational.org/ceta-information. Accessed May 27, 2022.
10. IEST. IEST-RP-CC034.4: HEPA and ULPA Filter Leak Tests. October 2009.
11. Controlled Environment Testing Association. CAG-003-2006-13. Certification of Sterile Compounding Facilities for USP Compliance. 2022.
12. NSF International. NSF/ANSI 49-2019. Biosafety Cabinetry: Design, Construction, Performance, And Field Certification. 2019.
13. Controlled Environment Testing Association. CAG-002-2006. CETA Compounding Isolator Testing Guide. December 8, 2008.

UNIT 3

Summary: Facilities and Engineering Controls

Definition Overview

Segregated Compounding Area (SCA)	Designated spaces or rooms in which a PEC may be placed for the preparation of non-hazardous, Category 1 CSPs
Clean room suite	A classified area that consists of both an anteroom and buffer room for compounding Category 2 and 3 CSPs
Buffer room	An ISO Class 7 or cleaner room with fixed walls and doors where PEC(s) are physically located. It may only be accessed through the anteroom or another buffer room.
Anteroom	An ISO Class 8 or cleaner room with fixed walls and doors where personnel hand hygiene, garbing procedures, and other particle generating activities. It is the transition room between the unclassified area and the buffer room.
Air changes per hour (ACPH)	The number of times the air fully exchanges in a room. It is how room airflow is measured.
LAFW	Laminar airflow workbench
IVLFZ	Integrated vertical laminar flow zone
CAI	Compounding aseptic isolator
BSC	Biological safety cabinet
CACI	Compounding aseptic containment isolator

SCA and Cleanroom Suite Summary Comparison

SCA	Clean Room Suite
Unclassified	ISO-Classified • ISO 7 buffer room • ISO 7 or 8 anteroom
HEPA-filtration not required	HEPA-filtration
ACPH not required	Buffer room ACPH requirements • 30 ACPH • At least 15 ACPH from the HVAC system Anteroom ACPH requirements • 20 ACPH • At least 15 ACPH from the HVAC system
No pressure requirements*	Pressure requirements • 0.020-inches water column between each ISO area • 0.020-inches water column between the anteroom and unclassified space
Comfortable work conditions	Recommended temperature and humidity • 20°C or cooler • Relative humidity of less than 60%
Perimeter line that defines the SCA	Line of demarcation to separate the clean and dirty sides of the anteroom

*Containment segregated compounding areas (C-SCAs) do have pressure requirements.

PEC Comparison

PEC	Airflow	Use	Location	
			Category 1	Category 2 or 3
LAFW	Horizontal or Vertical	Non-hazardous	SCA	ISO Class and buffer room with ISO Class 7 or 8 anteroom
IVLFZ	Vertical	Non-hazardous	N/A	
CAI	Vertical	Non-hazardous	SCA	
BSC	Vertical	Non-hazardous or hazardous	SCA	
CACI	Vertical	Hazardous	SCA	
Isolator	Vertical	Non-hazardous or hazardous	SCA	ISO Class 8 positive pressure room

Certification Comparison

Clean Room Suite	LAFW	BSC	RABS
Airflow testing	Airflow/Velocity testing	Airflow/Velocity testing	Airflow/Velocity testing
HEPA filter integrity testing	HEPA filter integrity testing	HEPA filter integrity testing	HEPA filter integrity testing
Total particle count testing	Total particle count testing	Total particle count testing	Total particle count testing
Room segregation (pressure differential)	Dynamic airflow smoke pattern test	Dynamic airflow smoke pattern test	Dynamic airflow smoke pattern test
Visual smoke study	Induction leak/ backstreaming test	Intake velocity and inflow volume	Chamber pressure test
Temperature and humidity		Site installation assessment	Ingress and egress test
		Airflow containment verification	Particle containment test (CACI only)
			Site installation assessment (CACI only)

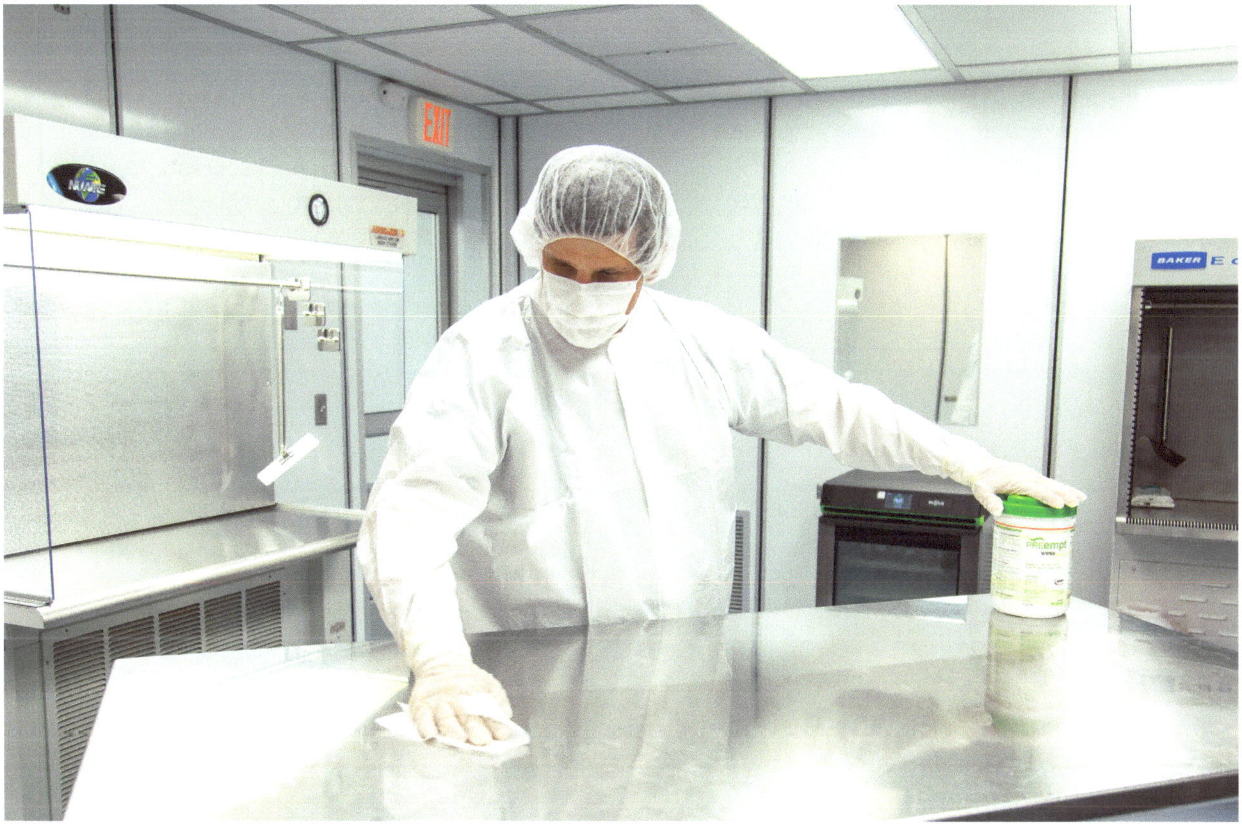

Photo courtesy of Contec, Inc.

UNIT 4

Maintenance of the Clean Room

Usually, when someone thinks of cleaning, visions of vacuum cleaners, mops, dusters, and bottles of chemicals come to mind. Cleaning a sterile compounding environment is very different than cleaning a home, office, or even a hospital room. Because of this, specialized tools, cleaning materials, and training are essential. The cleaning and disinfection of a sterile compounding facility is very complex and requires those overseeing and performing the task to have a thorough understanding of cleaning concepts and an appreciation for why these activities are so important. In this unit we will explore the concepts of cleaning and identify USP <797> requirements and practical solutions for the maintenance of sterile compounding environments.

Cleaning-Related Definitions

To understand the process of cleaning, one must understand cleaning-related terms. The important terms used by USP General Chapter <797> include cleaning, cleaning agent, disinfection, disinfectant, sporicidal disinfectant, 1-step disinfectant cleaner, and contact. Another important term that is not defined in USP <797> is sanitize.

Have you heard these cleaning terms before? How do you apply these terms to cleaning activities at your organization?

Cleaning and Cleaning Agent

USP <797> defines cleaning as "the process of removing substances (e.g., organic and inorganic material) from objects and surfaces, normally accomplished by manually or mechanically using water with detergents or enzymatic products."[1] This definition indicates that a detergent or cleaner must be used to remove the soil load from a surface to allow for further action. What does "further action" mean? For sterile compounding purposes, the appropriate further action would be disinfection. It is important to note that in the CDC definition, the term decontamination is used to address bloodborne pathogens, not hazardous drug decontamination.

USP <797> provides a definition for cleaning agent: "An agent for the removal of residues (e.g., dirt, debris, microbes, and residual drugs or chemicals) from surfaces."[1] Notice that it only mentions the removal from surfaces and not the ability to destroy or kill microorganisms. It is entirely possible that the cleaning agent could kill microorganisms, but the focus of the cleaning agent is to remove dirt, also known as a soil load. This is important because for a disinfectant to be effective, the surface must first be clean.

Based on these definitions we can summarize that cleaning is a mechanical process using detergent to remove dirt, residues, and microorganisms from a surface to prepare that surface for disinfection.

> **Did you know that sterile 70% IPA is not a cleaning agent?** It does not contain a detergent to remove dirt, so it is categorized as a disinfectant. However, for sterile IPA to be considered a disinfectant, it needs a 5-minute dwell time.[2] This is very difficult to achieve in a sterile compounding area without rewetting the surface. Therefore, we use sterile 70% IPA as a sanitizer. Anytime sterile 70% IPA is used; it must be allowed to dry to be effective. It is also an excellent residue remover.

Disinfection and Disinfectant

The CDC does provide definitions for both disinfection and disinfectant.[3]

Disinfection: Thermal or chemical destruction of pathogenic and other types of microorganisms. Disinfection is less lethal than sterilization because it destroys most recognized pathogenic microorganisms but not necessarily all microbial forms (e.g., bacterial spores).

Disinfectant: Usually a chemical agent (but sometimes a physical agent) that destroys disease-causing pathogens or other harmful microorganisms but might not kill bacterial spores. It refers to substances applied to inanimate objects.

USP <797> provides a definition for disinfectant. "A chemical or physical agent used on inanimate surfaces and objects to destroy fungi, viruses, and bacteria. Sporicidal disinfectants are considered a special class of disinfectants that also are effective against bacterial and fungal spores."[1] This definition indicates that certain disinfectants can be used against spores.

The chapter also mentions the use of a sporicidal disinfectant. This is "a chemical or physical agent that destroys bacterial and fungal spores when used in sufficient concentration for a specified contact time. It is expected to kill all vegetative microorganisms."[1]

When you hear the term disinfection, think of a chemical process that kills microorganisms, but not their spores. Only disinfection with a sporicidal disinfectant can destroy spores. The U.S. Environmental Protection Agency (EPA) oversees the designation of agents as disinfectants. To be a categorized as a disinfectant and have certain label claims, such as being sporicidal, the disinfectant must undergo rigorous testing.

> Remember, before performing disinfection, ask yourself if the surface was already cleaned with an agent that contains a detergent.

1-Step Disinfectant Cleaner

As was mentioned, it's not possible to effectively disinfect a surface until it's clean. But who wants to apply 2 different agents to a surface? Fortunately, there are agents available that, in the presence of a light to moderate soil load, can clean and disinfect in 1 application. USP <797> defines a 1-step disinfectant cleaner as "a product with an EPA-registered (or equivalent) claim that it can clean and disinfect a non-porous surface in the presence of light to moderate organic soiling without a separate cleaning step."[1] Think about the compounding environment. It's not common to see heavy, visible dirt or debris on surfaces. For that reason, 1-step disinfectant cleaning agents are perfect for sterile compounding surfaces.

To avoid having to separately clean and disinfect surfaces in the sterile compounding environment, use a 1-step disinfectant cleaner. Use an agent that is registered with the EPA, which ensures it is has been rigorously tested against a variety of microorganisms and that the contact times of the agent have been validated. Look to have both a bactericidal and sporicidal 1-step disinfectant cleaner available for your cleaning procedures.

Cleaning Up the Confusion:

Terminal Clean, Monthly Clean, and Triple Clean

The terms terminal clean, monthly clean, and triple clean are commonly inappropriately interchanged. Many sterile compounding organizations, especially those in a hospital, call their monthly clean a terminal clean or think that a triple clean and monthly clean are the same. A terminal clean is very different than the monthly clean performed in a sterile compounding facility and triple cleans are different yet.

The CDC defines a terminal cleaning as "cleaning and disinfection after the patient is discharged or transferred. Includes the removal of organic material and significant reduction and elimination of microbial contamination."[4] While USP does not have an official definition of a monthly clean, this is the sporicidal application to all surfaces in the clean room suite or SCA. This is a one-time application if a one-step sporicidal disinfectant cleaner is used.

The term triple clean, or 3-time clean, is not to be confused with the monthly clean. A triple clean is the cleaning of the target surface 3 times.[5] This term is not mentioned in USP <797> and is a cleaning principle that comes from aseptic manufacturing. Some state boards of pharmacy may require a triple clean post construction or when remediating an extreme microbial excursion. Typically, a triple clean is accomplished by applying a 1-step bactericidal disinfectant cleaner, followed by 2 applications of a 1-step sporicidal disinfectant cleaner. Exhibit 1 provides a summary of the terms terminal clean, monthly clean, and triple clean.

Practical Solution: *Although a triple clean is not required by USP <797>, consideration should be given to implementing it into your cleaning procedures. A triple clean in the SEC after construction or on a new piece of equipment, like a PEC, that is brought into the SEC can significantly reduce the microbial contamination and help ensure a microbial state of control.*

Exhibit 1

Summary of Commonly Misused Cleaning-Related Terms

Term	Where it applies	Required by	What it is	Agent
Terminal Clean	Patient room	CDC	Cleaning and disinfection of an area after patient discharge or transfer	Cleaner and disinfectant, may be 1-step depending on needs
Monthly Clean	SEC	USP <797>	Cleaning and application of a sporicidal disinfectant to all surfaces in the clean room or SCA	Cleaner and sporicidal disinfectant or a 1-step sporicidal disinfectant cleaner
Triple Clean	SEC	None – may be required by some state BOPs	3 applications of agents to prepare an area of item use or to remediate an extreme microbial excursion	1 application of a 1-step bactericidal disinfectant cleaner, followed by 2 applications of a 1-step sporicidal disinfectant cleaner

Contact Time

USP <797> mentions the term contact time but does not specifically define it. Contact time is also known as dwell time. The CDC defines dwell time as the "time a disinfectant is in direct contact with the surface or item to be disinfected. For surface disinfection, this period is framed by the application to the surface until complete drying has occurred."[3] Meeting the contact time is necessary to achieve the intended effect of the agent. Do you know the contact times of your cleaning agents?

The agent's label can be confusing because it likely lists multiple contact times, based on the desired outcome: achieving bacterial, fungicidal, or sporicidal activity. It's important to know what you are trying to achieve with an agent. All contact times should be documented in the organization's SOPs and staff need to be trained on the contact time of each agent.

Sanitize

Sanitize is not a term you will find in USP <797>; however, clean room personnel sanitize surfaces multiple times a day in the sterile compounding environment. A sanitizer is "an agent for reducing, on inanimate surfaces, the number of all forms of microbial life including fungi, viruses, and bacteria."[2] Think about how you use sterile 70% IPA. It's used after you have already cleaned and disinfected a surface, likely with a 1-step disinfectant cleaner. It is also used to further reduce the microorganisms on gloves, work surfaces, and even critical sites.

Importance of Cleaning

USP <797> very generally speaks to the importance of the cleaning process, indicating that surfaces are a potential source of CSP contamination and that cleaning, disinfecting, and applying a sporicidal disinfectant is important to address this contamination. While this is true, it is a very simple outlook on the criticality of cleaning. Cleaning goes hand in hand with a contamination control program. Although you might not specifically think of facility design, hand hygiene and garbing, material handling, and aseptic behaviors as part of a contamination control program, they are the key elements that keep microbial contamination from entering the compounding area. However, no matter how good a contamination control program is, some microorganisms will enter the compounding area. This is why cleaning is so important. Cleaning is the safety net to mitigate microbial contamination and protect patients.

> Be sure that all who have cleaning responsibilities in your facility understand the importance of cleaning as it relates to sterile compounding.

Cleaning Agents and Supplies

Choosing Agents

There are several things to consider when choosing agents for cleaning the sterile compounding area. Let's look at some questions you should ask when choosing an agent and why asking these questions is important.[6]

Is the agent an EPA-registered one-step disinfectant cleaner?

Using a 1-step disinfectant cleaner will shorten the cleaning time, because you can apply a single agent to clean and disinfect in 1 application. This will also aid in cleaning procedure compliance. The simpler the process, the more likely staff are to comply.

Does the agent have efficacy against the category of microorganisms you need to kill?

When it comes to disinfectants, it is important to know which microorganisms are destroyed by the agent. You may see disinfectants labeled as bactericidal, fungicidal, viricidal, and sporicidal. Sterile compounding facilities need to have available a 1-step bactericidal disinfectant cleaner for daily cleaning and a 1-step sporicidal disinfectant cleaner for weekly and monthly cleaning.

Does it come sterile?

USP <797> requires the use of a sterile agent to clean and disinfect the PEC. The chapter goes on to indicate that sterile agents should be used to clean classified areas.[1] There is no mention of using sterile cleaning agents to clean the SCA.

Does it come in a ready-to-use (RTU) formula?

Agents can come concentrated, where you add water, or ready-to-use (RTU). Choosing an RTU agent eliminates the preparation step, which can result in an improperly prepared agent. Overdiluted agents will not work as prescribed on the label. Underdiluted agents can leave excessive residue on surfaces. If you do choose to use a concentrate, you must use sterile water to prepare any agent used in the PEC and the preparation must be documented.

Is it compatible with the surfaces in the compounding area and other agents used?

Some agents may be incompatible with facility materials and cause rusting or corrosion, which is an insanitary condition according to the FDA.[7] There is also a risk that 2 agents may not be compatible with each other, causing a safety risk to staff. Be sure to review the manufactures' information for compatibility concerns.

Does it leave a residue?

Cleaning and disinfecting agents can leave residue, some more than others, and this residue can build up over time. Look for low-residue agents. If you are experiencing significant residue build up, consider implementing scheduled residue removal, using sterile water or sterile 70% IPA.[8]

Can the contact time be reasonably met?

To meet chapter requirements, the manufacturer's directions or published data for the minimum contact time must be followed for each of the cleaning, disinfecting, and sporicidal disinfectants used.[1] This seems simple enough, but airflow in the PEC and the clean room suite can make this difficult.[9] The constant air movement accelerates the drying rate, so agents with longer contact times might need to be applied multiple times to ensure the contact time is met. Look for agents with shorter contact times to avoid this issue.

Choosing Supplies

When choosing cleaning supplies, such as wipers, pads, and mopheads, USP <797> requires that they be low lint. This should also apply to tools, such as mop handles. The chapter has additional requirements for cleaning supplies.[1]

- Cleaning supplies, such as wipers, pads, and mopheads, used in the PEC must be sterile
- Tool handles and holders must be cleaned and disinfected prior to use in a PEC
- If disposable cleaning supplies are used, they must be discarded after each cleaning activity
- Reusable cleaning tools must be:
    - Made of cleanable materials
    - Cleaned and disinfected before and after each use
    - Dedicated for use in the classified areas or SCA
    - Kept in the dedicated area except for disposal
    - Discarded as determined based on the condition of the tools
- Mops used in areas where HDs are compounded must be dedicated for use only in those areas
- Cleaning supplies used in the classified areas and SCAs must be disposed of in a manner that minimizes the potential for dispersing contaminants into the air

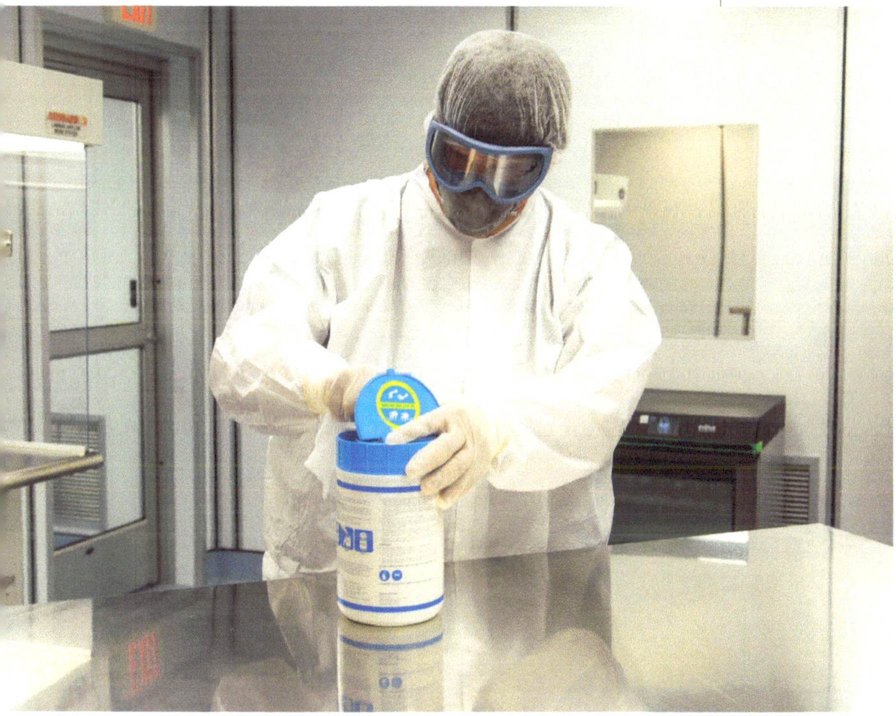

Photo courtesy of Contec, Inc.

Opened Sterile Cleaning Supplies

You use sterile cleaning supplies every day, like the bottles of sterile 70% IPA or sterile wipers presaturated with IPA. Have you defined in your SOPs the timeframe in which these items must be used once opened? USP <797> does not specify time, but instead leaves it to the organization to define in its SOPs. If you are not sure where to start, reach out to the manufacturer of the sterile product.

Clean to Dirty and High to Low Cleaning Principles

Cleaning in the right direction ensures that dirt and microorganisms will not drip, fall through, or be pulled through areas that have already been cleaned.

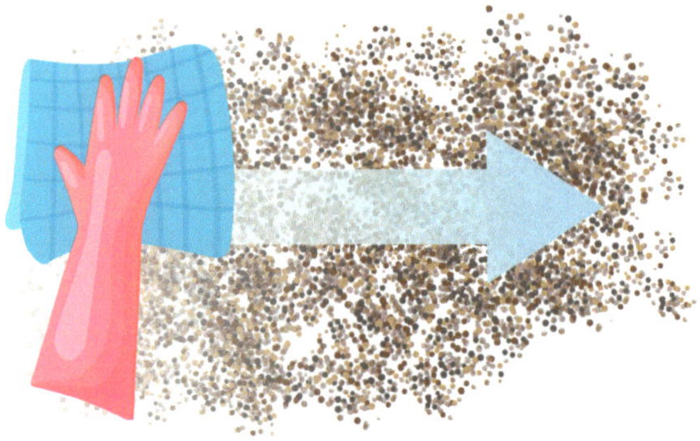

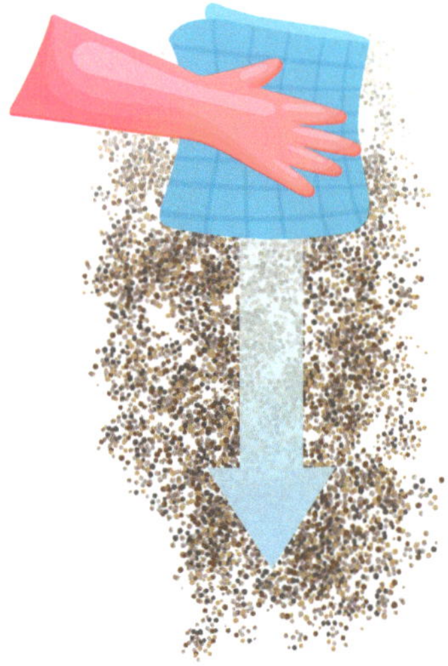

Practical Solution: *According to the chapter, wipers, pads, and mop heads used to clean the SEC* ***should be*** *disposable. This leaves it open for organizations to use reusable supplies. However, the chapter does not provide guidance on how the reusable item is expected to be maintained or laundered for reuse. It is best to utilize disposable cleaning supplies for both the PEC and the SEC. This greatly reduces the risk of contamination and avoids any confusion on where disposable or reusable supplies can be used.*

Cleaning Principles

The chapter indicates that cleaning must be performed in the direction of clean to dirty areas.[1] Clean to dirty can be hard to define. Think about a horizontal flow PEC. The HEPA filter is on the back wall of the device. Because of this, it could be argued that the back wall is the cleanest surface in the PEC, because of the airflow direction. But we also know there could be splashes and sprays of medication on the HEPA filter screen, which could take this surface out of the running for the cleanest surface. We also need to think about the cleaning principle of cleaning from high to low (top to bottom). This technique prevents "dirt and microorganisms from dripping or falling and contaminating already cleaned areas."[10] Therefore, based on this technique, it makes the most sense to start with the ceiling of the PEC. We'll discuss PEC cleaning order later in this unit.

If the cleaning order of a PEC is that complicated to determine, how is a clean room or SCA during a monthly clean best handled? Because there is no right way to clean a PEC, clean room, or SCA, the organization must determine a cleaning sequence best suited for their operation based on clean-to-dirty and high-to-low principles and document the order in their SOPs.[5]

Cleaning supplies also need to be used from clean to dirty. For example, a mop head used on the floor can be used to clean both the buffer room and anteroom, but the floor in the buffer room must be cleaned before the floor in the anteroom.

Wiping and Mopping Path

Have you heard that you need to use unidirectional overlapping strokes to clean? You won't find this language in USP <797>! However, this is the best technique to use for wiping and mopping surfaces.[11]

Even though the goal is to have easily cleanable, flat surfaces in the sterile compounding area, there are many irregular surfaces. These irregular surfaces present a cleaning challenge, as they cannot be cleaned using a flat tool or mop. Irregular surfaces need to be carefully cleaned by hand with wipers, being sure to saturate all surfaces for adequate agent contact time. Examples of irregular surfaces in the PEC are IV bars, hooks, and cups that hold the IV bar. There are a variety of irregular surfaces in the SEC including life safety signs, clocks, wall hooks, return grills, and the exterior of PECs. Include specific cleaning instructions for irregular surfaces in your SOPs and be sure those responsible for cleaning are trained on how to properly clean these surfaces.

Cleaning Frequency

USP <797> defines the cleaning frequency and the general agents used. Some cleaning activities are performed daily, while others are weekly or monthly based on the category of CSPs compounded. Remember that even if you compound in an SCA, the surfaces listed below within the perimeter of the SCA must still be cleaned.

PEC(s) and equipment inside the PEC(s)

- Cleaned and disinfected on days when compounding occurs or when surface contamination is known or suspected
- Sanitized with sterile 70% IPA after cleaning and disinfection and at least every 30 minutes
- Sporicidal disinfectant application monthly for Category 1 and 2, weekly for Category 3

PEC removable work tray

- Cleaned and disinfected on days when compounding occurs
- Sanitized with sterile 70% IPA after cleaning and at least every 30 minutes
- Sporicidal disinfectant application monthly Area under the PEC removable work tray
- Cleaned and disinfected monthly
- Sanitized with sterile 70% IPA monthly
- Sporicidal disinfectant application monthly

Pass-through chambers, work surfaces outside the PEC, and floors

- Cleaned and disinfected on days when compounding occurs
- Sporicidal disinfectant application monthly for Category 1 and 2, weekly for Category 3

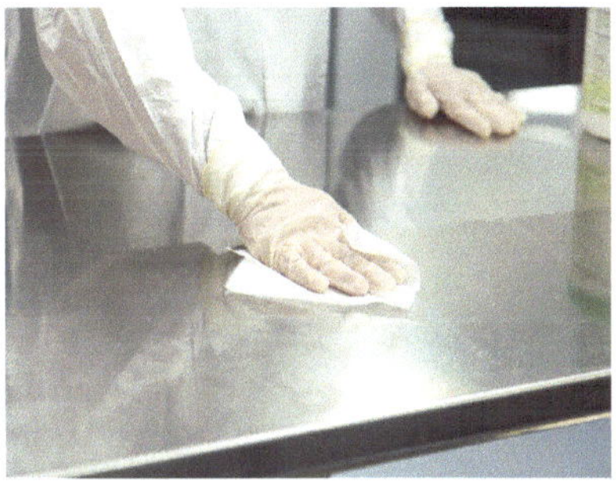

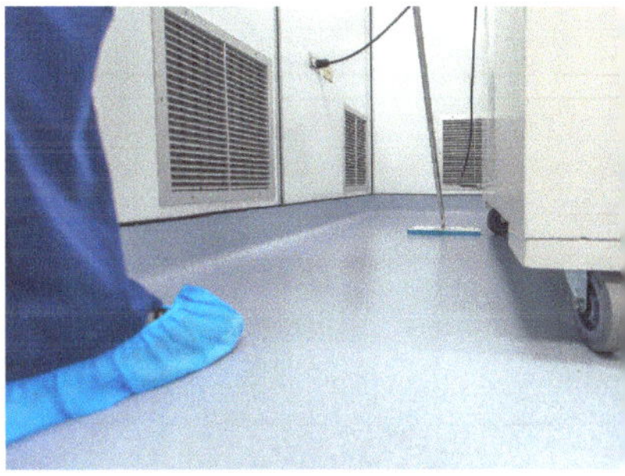

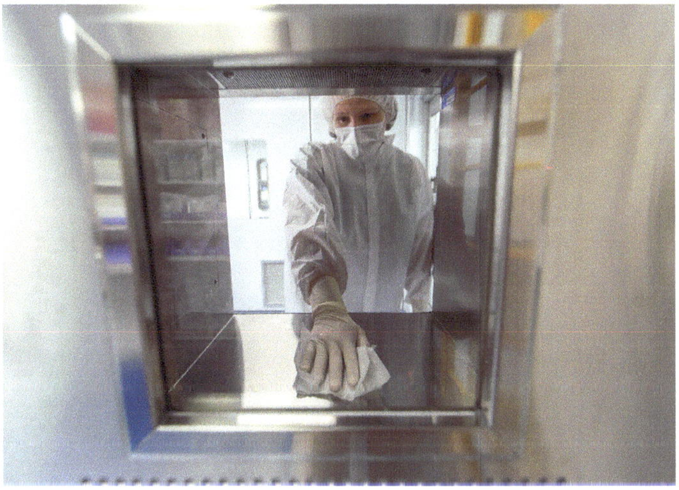

Photos courtesy of Contec, Inc.

Surfaces of the sink

- Cleaned and disinfected each day of use
- Sporicidal disinfectant application at least monthly

Equipment outside the PEC, including the exteriors of the PECs

- Cleaned and disinfected monthly
- Sporicidal disinfectant application monthly

Walls, doors, door frames, ceilings, storage shelving, bins, and anything else in the SEC

- Cleaned and disinfected monthly
- Sporicidal disinfectant application monthly

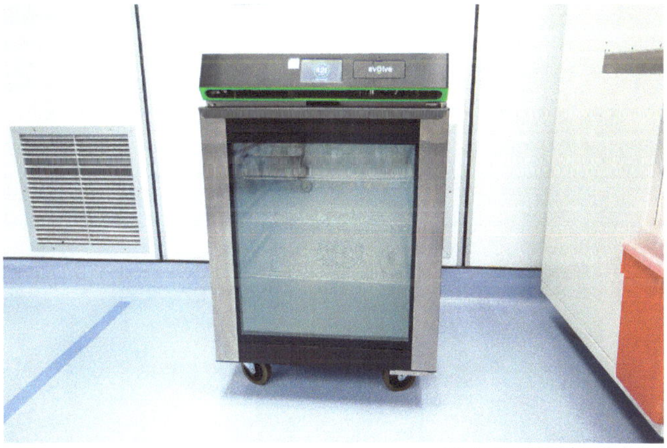

Photo courtesy of Contec, Inc.

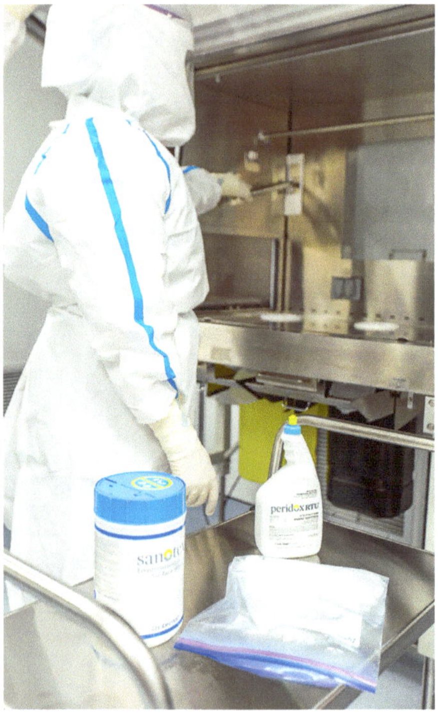

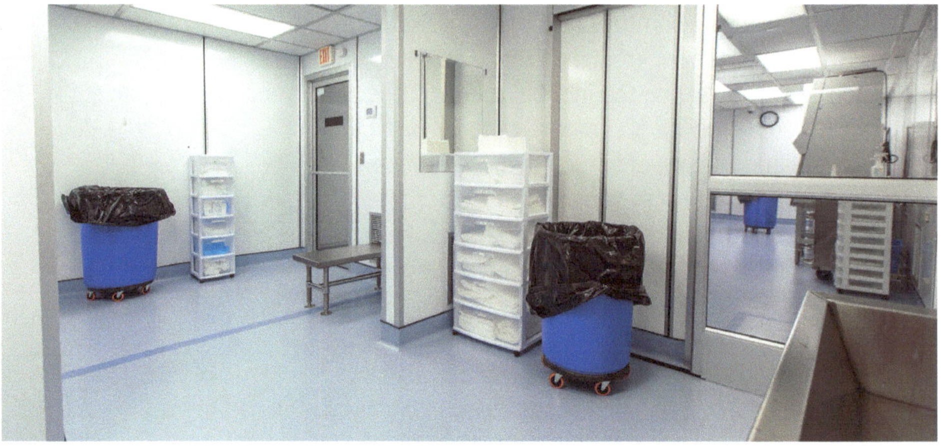

Photos courtesy of Contec, Inc.

Exhibit 2 summarizes the cleaning required in the clean room suite and the segregated compounding area on the daily, weekly, and monthly basis. It also provides some practical solutions to assist with contamination control.

Exhibit 2

SEC Cleaning Frequency Summary

Daily	Weekly	Monthly
Cleaning and disinfection, ideally with a 1-step bactericidal disinfectant cleaner	Cleaning and sporicidal disinfectant application, ideally with a 1-step sporicidal disinfectant cleaner	
USP Requirement • Work surfaces outside PEC • Pass-through chambers • Floors • Sinks **Practical Solution** • High-touch surfaces • Staging cart	**Category 3 USP Requirement** • Work surfaces outside PEC • Pass-through chambers • Floors **Category 1 and 2 Practical Solution** • Same surfaces as the in the daily column	**USP Requirement** • Work surfaces outside PEC • Pass-through chambers • Sinks • Floors and ceilings • Walls, doors, door frames • Storage shelving and bins • Equipment outside PEC **Practical Solution** • EVERYTHING in the SEC

Cleaning the PEC

Proper PEC cleaning is essential to a successful contamination control strategy. The technique and agents used are what ensure successful removal of contamination from PEC surfaces. At a minimum the cleaning of the PEC will require the application of 2 agents. But it could be more depending on the agents used. Exhibit 3 defines the types of agents used to clean the PEC and the order of application, based on whether 1-step disinfectant agents are chosen.

USP <797> provides instructions on how to clean and disinfect the PEC, as well as how to apply a sporicidal disinfectant. The first step in cleaning the PEC is to remove visible particles, debris, or residue with an

Exhibit 3

Order of Agent Application to Clean the PEC Based on Agents Used

Cleaning and Disinfection		Applying Sporicidal Disinfectant	
If you use separate cleaning and disinfecting agents, cleaning the PEC will require application of 3 agents.	If you use a 1-step disinfectant cleaner, cleaning the PEC will require application of 2 agents.	If you use a separate cleaning and sporicidal disinfecting agents	If you use a 1-step sporicidal disinfectant cleaner
1. Cleaning agent 2. Disinfecting agent 3. Sterile 70% IPA	1. 1-step disinfectant cleaner 2. Sterile 70% IPA	1. Cleaning agent 2. Sporicidal disinfectant. 3. Sterile 70% IPA	1. 1-step sporicidal disinfectant cleaner 2. Sterile 70% IPA

Exhibit 4

Cleaning and Disinfecting the PEC

Chapter Requirement[2]	Real-life Practice
Cleaning and Disinfecting the PEC	
Remove visible particles, debris, or residue with an appropriate solution (e.g., Sterile Water for Injection or Sterile Water for Irrigation) using sterile, low-lint wipers	It is unlikely that there will be visible particles, debris, or residue in the PEC. This means you do not need to use sterile water every time the PEC is cleaned. Be sure SOPs indicate how the organization handles visible contamination.
Using a sterile, low-lint wiper, apply a sterile cleaning agent followed by a sterile disinfecting agent or apply an EPA-registered (or equivalent) 1-step disinfectant cleaner to equipment and all interior surfaces of the PEC	Apply a sterile, 1-step disinfectant cleaner to equipment and all interior surfaces of the PEC using a sterile, low-lint wiper or cleaning tool.
Ensure the contact time specified by the manufacturer is achieved	Be sure the contact time is met.
Using a sterile, low-lint wiper, apply sterile 70% IPA to equipment and all interior surfaces in the PEC	Apply sterile 70% IPA to equipment and all interior surfaces of the PEC using a sterile, low-lint wiper or cleaning tool.
Allow the surface to dry completely before beginning compounding	Allow the surface to dry completly before transferring any items into the PEC.
Applying a Sporicidal Disinfectant in the PEC	
Remove visible particles, debris, or residue with an appropriate solution (e.g., Sterile Water for Injection or Sterile Water for Irrigation) using sterile, low-lint wipers	It is unlikely that there will be visible particles, debris, or residue in the PEC. This means you do not need to use sterile water every time the PEC is cleaned. Be sure you SOP indicates how your organization handles visible contamination.
After cleaning and disinfecting, apply the sterile sporicidal disinfectant using a sterile, low-lint wiper to all surfaces and the area underneath the work tray; if the sporicidal disinfectant is an EPA-registered (or equivalent) 1-step disinfectant sporicidal cleaner, separate cleaning and disinfecting steps are not required	Apply a 1-step sporicidal disinfectant cleaner to equipment, all interior surfaces of the PEC, and the area underneath the work tray using a sterile, low-lint wiper or cleaning tool.
Ensure the contact time specified by the manufacturer is achieved	Be sure the contact time is met.
Using a sterile low-lint wiper, apply sterile 70% IPA to all interior surfaces, including underneath the work tray	Apply sterile 70% IPA to equipment, all interior surfaces of the PEC, and underneath the work tray using a sterile, low-lint wiper or cleaning tool.
Allow the surface to dry completely before beginning compounding	Allow the surface to dry before transferring any items into the PEC.

appropriate solution. The chapter provides sterile water for injection or sterile water for irrigation as examples of what could be used.[1] Note that this is only required if there is visible contamination, which will not be every time you clean, and you don't have to use sterile water. Another option would be to use a 1-step disinfectant cleaner once to remove the visible contamination and then again as the cleaning and disinfection step. However you decide to manage the requirement of removing visible contamination, be sure it is documented in your SOPs.

The next step is to apply a sterile cleaning agent followed by a sterile disinfecting agent, using a sterile, low-lint wiper to all interior PEC surfaces and equipment. Alternatively, you could apply a 1-step disinfectant cleaner. It is difficult to reach all surfaces of the PEC interior without needing to lean into the PEC. To avoid this insanitary condition, consider using a cleaning tool.[7] Be sure the contact time of the agent is met.[7]

The last step is to apply sterile 70% IPA to equipment and all interior surfaces in the PEC, using a sterile low-lint wiper. This step further sanitizes the surfaces and removes any cleaning agent residue. The sterile 70% IPA must be allowed to dry before beginning any compounding activities.

Exhibit 4 reviews these steps and provides insight into real-life cleaning practices.

The chapter's direction on applying a sporicidal disinfectant to the PEC is like that of cleaning and disinfection. There are 2 small differences. First, the chapter specifically indicates that the sporicidal disinfectant and sterile 70% IPA must be applied to the area under the PEC work tray if one exists. This applies to BSCs, CAIs, and CACIs. Second, the chapter does not specify in Box 8 like it does in Box 7 that equipment in the PEC needs to have sporicidal disinfectant applied. However, it is indicated in Table 10 that sporicidal agents are to be applied to the equipment contained in the PEC. To ensure a microbial state of control in the PEC, apply a sporicidal disinfectant to equipment as well. Review both the equipment and disinfectant manufacturers' instructions for use for compatibility concerns.

Even though there is cleaning guidance from USP <797>, the chapter does not specifically define the cleaning order of surfaces in the PEC. In remembering the clean-to-dirty and high-to-low cleaning principles, a generally accepted cleaning order can be identified, as shown in Exhibit 5. However, it is up to the organization to define its specific cleaning order in its SOPs.

As part of routine PEC use during the compounding day, USP <797> requires that sterile 70% IPA be applied to the work surface at least every 30 minutes if the compounding process takes 30 minutes or less. If the compounding process takes longer than 30 minutes, compounding is not disrupted, and the work surface is wiped with sterile 70% IPA immediately after compounding.[1] This frequent sanitization of the PEC work surface is valuable in reducing the microbial contamination in the PEC.

Cleaning the SEC

Other than cleaning frequency and agents to be used, USP <797> does not specifically address cleaning order or techniques for the SEC. The principles of cleaning discussed previously apply to both the cleaning of the clean room suite and within the perimeter of the SCA. For example, the daily cleaning of the clean room suite should move from the buffer to the anteroom. In deciding order for the SEC monthly cleaning, you could clean ceiling to floor in the buffer room, doing the PECs last, or start in the PECs and then do ceiling to floor, working your way out to the anteroom. Consider doing irregular surfaces by hand first and then using cleaning tools for flat surfaces.

Training, Documentation, and SOPs

Who performs cleaning in your organization? Are sterile compounding staff responsible for all the cleaning? Is some outsourced? How do you ensure outsourced staff are trained?

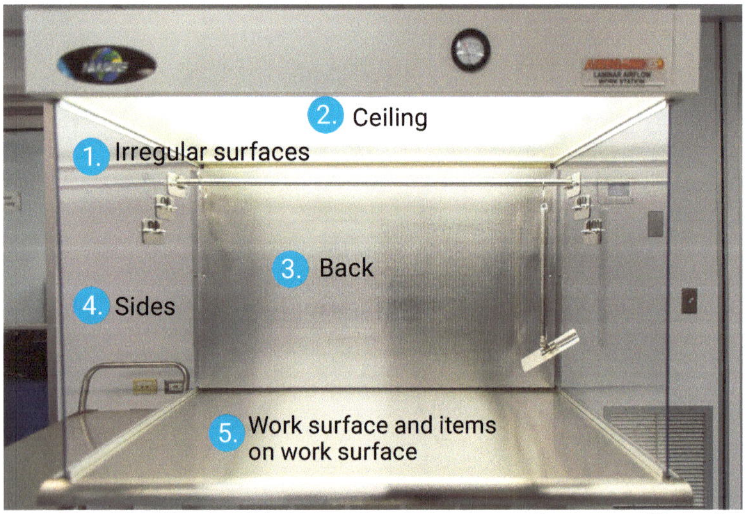

Photo courtesy of Contec, Inc.

There is no right or wrong when it comes to who cleans the sterile compounding area, but anyone who does must be trained on facility SOPs. Tracking the training of sterile compounding staff is much easier than tracking the training of outsourced staff. If you choose to outsource cleaning responsibilities, be sure you have training records on file for all individuals who enter to clean the sterile compounding area. The sterile compounding facility is responsible for their training in regards to cleaning protocols and SOPs, not their employer. All personnel with any cleaning responsibilities must be trained if there are any changes in the cleaning procedures. Compounders, designated persons, and those with direct oversight of compounding

Exhibit 5
Generally accepted cleaning order for a PEC

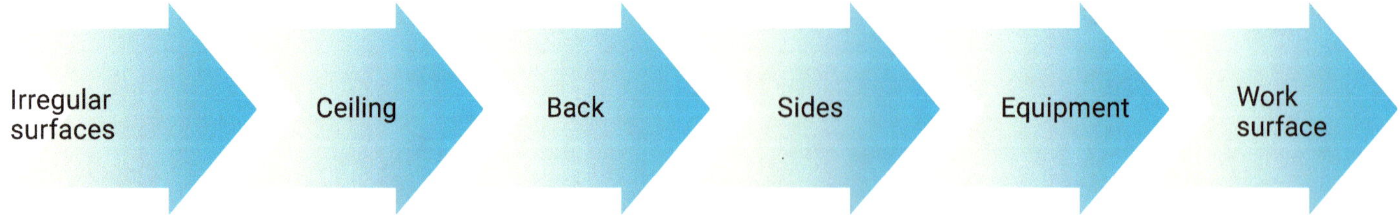

The current version of the chapter does not mention whether you can clean while compounding takes place. However, the 2008 version did indicate that floors in the buffer room, anteroom, and SCA must be cleaned when no aseptic operations are taking place. This is a good practice to follow not only for the cleaning of floors but for any cleaning activity that could increase the number of particles in the compounding area.

Practical Solution: Consider frequent sanitization of high-touch surfaces throughout the compounding day. Contamination risk points like touch screens, workflow management systems, pass-throughs, work surfaces outside the PEC, and other high-touch surfaces should be sanitized frequently. This is in an effort to mitigate the microbial contamination introduced throughout the compounding day.

operations must be trained and demonstrate competency in cleaning activities initially and at least every 12 months. Pharmacy staff or external cleaning staff that are allowed to clean the interior of the PECs must be trained and demonstrate competency in cleaning activities initially and at least every 12 months. Pharmacy staff or external cleaning staff that are NOT allowed to clean the interior of the PECs must be trained and demonstrate competency in cleaning activities initially and at a frequency defined by facility SOPs.

Practical Solution: *Although not specified in USP <797>, it is best to only allow sterile compounding personnel to clean the PEC. They understand how critical the ISO Class 5 area is to patient safety.*

USP <797> has specific requirements for cleaning SOPs and documentation.[1]

- Facility-approved agents and procedures must be defined in SOPs.
- SOPs must contain the frequency, method(s), and location(s) of cleaning, disinfecting, and applying sporicidal disinfectants, in accordance with the manufacturer's instructions.
- Those performing any cleaning responsibilities must follow all SOPs.
- Changes in the cleaning and disinfecting procedures require personnel training.
- All cleaning, disinfecting, and application of sporicidal disinfectants must be documented according to the facility's SOPs.

The chapter allows for the organization to make a lot of its own decisions on the cleaning process, based on its unique organizational needs and operations. Inspectors and surveyors will inevitably ask why you made the decisions you did. Capture in your SOPs or in a supporting document to show the rationale for the decisions made.

Summary

Cleaning is an essential part of a sterile compounding operation. It is more than just wiping and mopping. Sterile compounding personnel who take part in cleaning must understand the importance of their task and be focused on impeccable performance. Daily PEC and SEC cleaning aids in the maintenance of a low bioburden environment, while the weekly and monthly sporicidal disinfectant applications eliminate difficult-to-eradicate microorganisms. Construct cleaning SOPs that meet the organization's unique needs and ensure they are followed by all for consistent microbial control.

References

1. United States Pharmacopeia. <797> Pharmaceutical Compounding—Sterile Preparations. Proposed Revision. September 2021.
2. Ecolab. Klercide™ 70/30 IPA - Blended with WFI Product Overview. July 2019.
3. Centers for Disease Control and Prevention. Glossary: Guideline for Disinfection and Sterilization in Healthcare Facilities. 2016.
4. Centers for Diseases Control and Prevention. Best Practices for Environmental Cleaning in Healthcare Facilities: in Resource-Limited Settings. Version 2.
5. Douglass, K., Roth, A. Part 1 – Principles that Drive Effective Cleaning. *Pharmacy Purchasing & Products*. March 2020 – Vol. 17 No. 3.
6. Roth, A. Agents for Cleaning and Disinfecting Sterile Compounding Areas. INFUSION.2022;28(3):45-50.
7. The Food and Drug Administration. Insanitary Conditions at Compounding Facilities: Guidance for Industry. November 2020.
8. Douglass, K., Roth, A. Part 2 – Practice to Drive Effective Cleaning. *Pharmacy Purchasing & Products*. June 2020 – Vol. 17 No. 6.
9. Douglass, K., Roth, A. Part 3 or 3 – Answers to Common Cleaning Questions. *Pharmacy Purchasing & Products*. September 2020 – Vol. 17 No. 9.
10. Center for Diseases Control and Prevention. Environmental Cleaning in Resource-Limited Settings. Chapter 4. Environmental Cleaning Procedures. Page Reviewed April 21, 2020.
11. Cleanroom Technology. Successful Wiping. November 21, 2011.

Summary: Cleaning and Disinfection

Definition Overview

Cleaning agent	Removes residues from surfaces, contains a detergent
Disinfectant	Destroys viruses, bacteria, and fungi, but not their spores
Sporicidal agent	Destroys bacterial and fungal spores
1-step disinfectant cleaner	Cleans and disinfects in 1 step, can be bactericidal or sporicidal
Sanitizer	Reduces, on inanimate surfaces, the number of fungi and bacteria
Triple clean	The cleaning of the target surface 3 times

This table showcases the real-life cleaning practices of PECs and SECs. It combines USP <797> requirements with practical solutions to provide a robust cleaning schedule. Note that the required Category 3 weekly cleaning requirements are recommended for all CSP categories.

	Daily on days when compounding occurs	Weekly	Monthly
Agent	• 1-step bactericidal disinfectant cleaner • In the PEC, follow with sterile 70% IPA	1-step sporicidal disinfectant cleaner	1-step sporicidal disinfectant cleaner
PEC	• Interior • Removable work tray • Equipment	• Interior • Removable work tray • Equipment	• Interior • Removable work tray • Under removable work tray • Equipment
SEC	• Work surfaces outside PEC • Pass-throughs • Floors • Sink • High-touch surfaces • Staging cart	• Work surfaces outside PEC • Pass-throughs • Floors • Sink • High-touch surfaces • Staging cart	• Every surface in the clean room suite or perimeter of the SCA • All compounding supplies

PEC Cleaning Steps for Both 1-step Bacteriacidal and Sporicidal Disinfectant Cleaner Application

1. Remove visible contamination according to facility procedures, if needed.
2. Apply a sterile, 1-step disinfectant cleaner to equipment and all interior surfaces of the PEC using a sterile, low-lint wiper or cleaning tool.
3. Be sure the contact time is met.
4. Apply sterile 70% IPA to equipment and all interior surfaces of the PEC using a sterile, low-lint wiper or cleaning tool.
5. Allow the surface to dry before transferring any items into the PEC.

For the monthly PEC cleaning, apply the 1-step sporicidal disinfectant cleaner under the work tray and follow with sterile 70% IPA.

PEC Cleaning Order

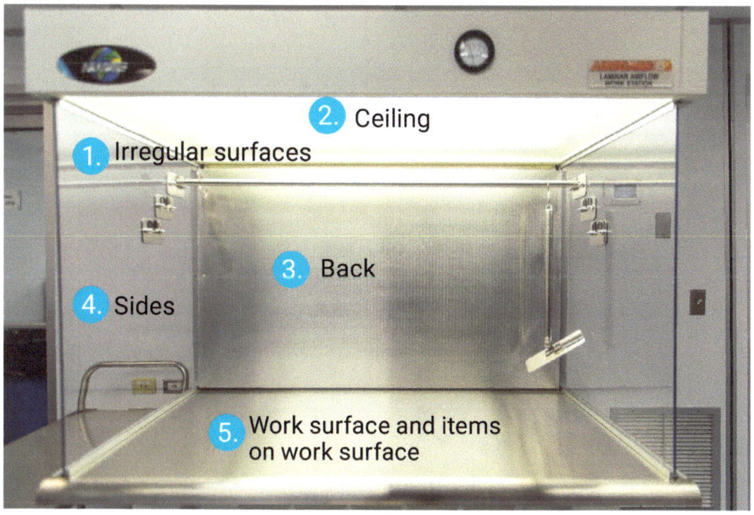

Photo courtesy of Contec, Inc.

General Cleaning Concepts and Tips

- Clean from cleanest to dirtiest and from high to low, as defined in your SOPs.
- If separate cleaning and disinfecting agents are used, cleaning must be performed before disinfection.
- Sterile 70% IPA is used in the sterile compounding environment as a sanitizer to reduce the number of microorganisms on surfaces.
- Terminal cleans are for patient care areas, not sterile compounding facilities.
- Sterile, disposable cleaning agents and supplies must be used in the PEC and should be used in the SEC. Disposable cleaning supplies (wipers, pads, mop heads) reduce the risk of contamination from reusable supplies.
- Document all cleaning activities, including the preparation of agents, if applicable.
- All staff, even those who are outsourced, must be trained and demonstrate competency in the tasks they perform every 12 months.
- Cease compounding while cleaning occurs.
- Document the rationale for the organization-specific decisions made regarding cleaning.

UNIT 5

Aseptic Practices

Have you ever really thought about how your movement, behavior, and actions in a compounding environment could potentially affect the sterility of CSPs, and thus, patient safety? You've likely been trained on what to do and how to behave, but do you know why these things are important? There is more to producing a safe CSP than donning proper garb and working in a PEC. Every action taken in and immediately outside the sterile compounding area could affect the microbial control of the clean room suite or SCA and ultimately the CSP. This unit defines aseptic technique, provides the whys behind the contamination control elements found in USP General Chapter <797>, and describes some practical solutions for aseptic practices.

What Is Aseptic Technique?

Until the latest version, USP <797> did not provide a definition of aseptic technique.[1] It seems impossible that a standard on sterile compounding would not define the one essential element critical to the production of a safe mediation. To temporarily fill a void, Sterile Compounding Educator Eric Kastango defined aseptic technique as *"a set of specific work practices and procedures performed under carefully controlled conditions with the goal of minimizing the introduction of contamination."*[2] In comparison, USP defines aseptic technique as *"a set of methods used to keep objects and areas free of microorganisms and thereby minimize infection risk to the patient. It is accomplished through practices that maintain the microbe count at an irreducible minimum."*[1]

Take a moment to think about what each of these definitions is really saying. How are they the same? How are they different?

The first thing you likely noticed is that both definitions indicate that there must be a defined way of doing things. There must be SOPs in place specific to the goal. Another similarity is that both are concerned with microbial contamination. This makes sense, as the

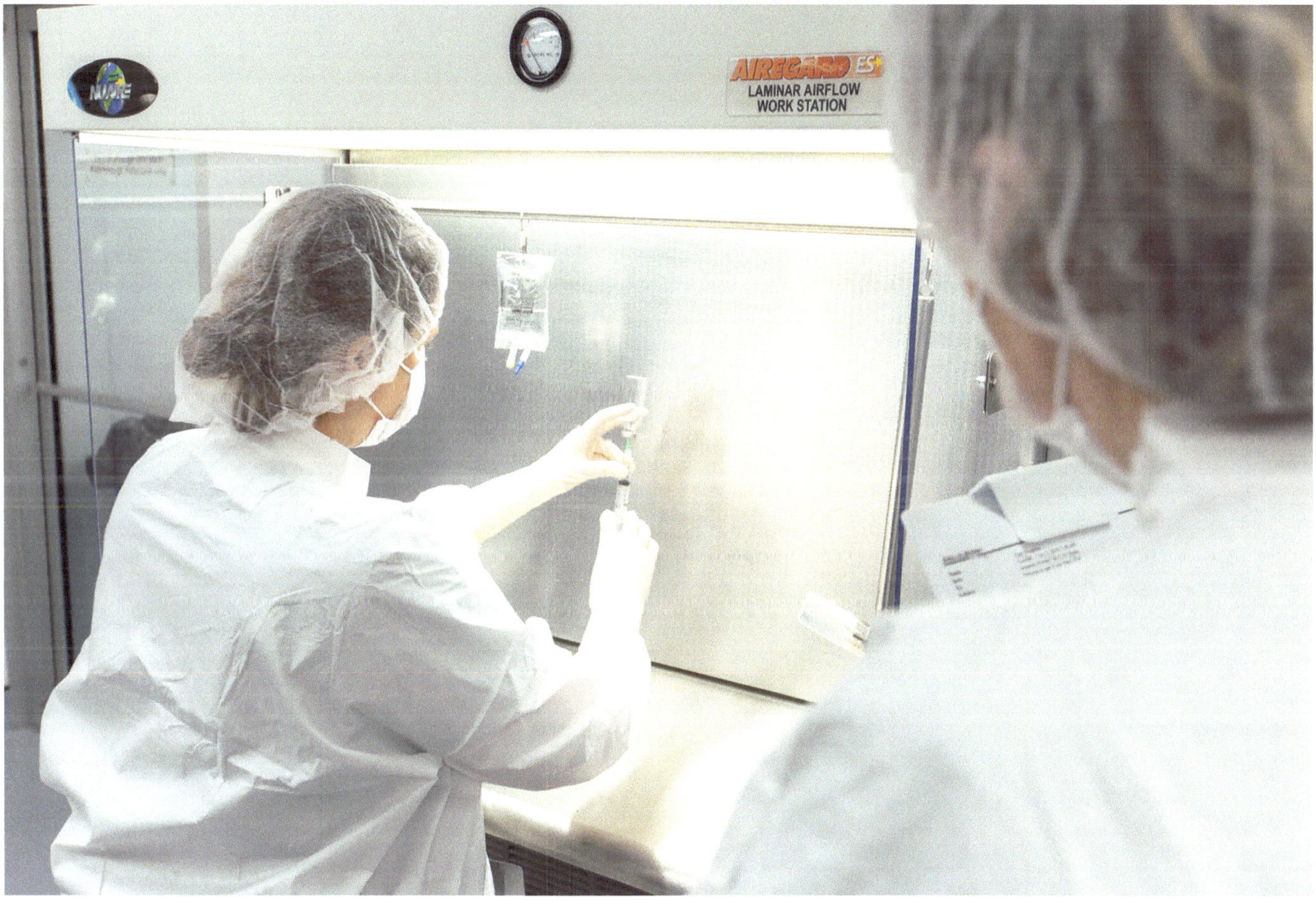

Photo courtesy of Contec, Inc.

medication prepared must be sterile. However, the definitions are slightly different when it comes to the expectation of microbial contamination. One has the goal of minimizing the introduction of contamination while the other focuses more on keeping objects and areas free of contamination. Although the difference may seem negligible, the former is more indicative of an actual sterile compounding operation, while the latter is an idealistic hope.

Based on the engineering controls, contamination control elements, and cleaning procedures required by USP <797> there will always be microorganisms in the sterile compounding environment. Even the most robust aseptic manufacturing environments recover microorganisms, and their facilities and procedures are well beyond the minimum requirements of the chapter. Keeping this mind, the goal should be to minimize microbial recovery as opposed to having zero recovery. Let's explore the contamination control elements and practical solutions that will facilitate reaching that goal.

Personal Hygiene

One of the most basic elements of contamination control is personal hygiene. Those working in the sterile compounding environment must maintain proper personal hygiene.[1] This is essential to minimize microbial contamination of the clean room suite and the SCA that is brought in on hair, skin, clothing, and shoes.

In the simplest terms, "personal hygiene refers to maintaining cleanliness of one's body and clothing to preserve overall health and wellbeing."[3] For sterile compounders the focus is on general cleanliness, clothing, hand hygiene, and nails.

There are some basic things personnel can do to help minimize microbial contamination. Be sure to include these in your SOPs.

1. Shower daily, preferably before the shift
2. Wear clean, laundered clothing
3. Wash hands[7]
   a. Before and after eating
   b. After using the restroom
   c. After blowing nose, coughing, or sneezing
4. Moisturize skin, especially face and arms[8]
5. Keep nails clean and neatly trimmed

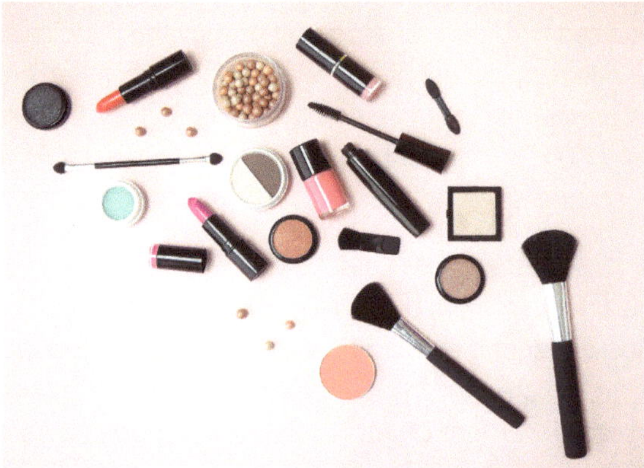

USP <797> also requires that all cosmetics be removed before entering the sterile compounding area.[1] The chapter does not define cosmetics, but FDA does. The agency defines cosmetics by their intended use, as *"articles intended to be rubbed, poured, sprinkled, or sprayed on, introduced into, or otherwise applied to the human body . . . for cleansing, beautifying, promoting attractiveness, or altering the appearance."* Among the products included in this definition are *"skin moisturizers,*

How People Introduce Bacteria to the Sterile Compounding Environment

Human skin is estimated to harbor ~10^{12} bacteria.[4] That's a trillion microorganisms, just on our skin! This wouldn't be too much of a concern if the average adult didn't lose close to 500 million skin cells a day.[5] When we shed those skin cells, we also shed bacteria. Skin shedding, along with aerosolization of oral and respiratory fluids, are the main sources of indoor airborne bacteria.[6]

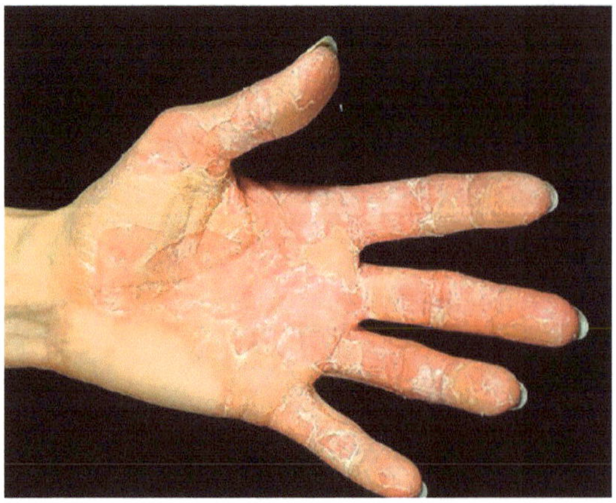

perfumes, lipsticks, fingernail polishes, eye and facial makeup preparations, cleansing shampoos, permanent waves, hair colors, and deodorants."[9] This definition includes essential products used for personal hygiene, which are necessary. Focus should be on the other products, such as make up and nail polish, which can flake particles. Specifically, the chapter requires that nails are kept clean and neatly trimmed and that nail products like polish, artificial nails, and extenders must not be worn.[1]

How can we moisturize? Isn't lotion a cosmetic? Yes, FDA considers lotion a cosmetic. But using untinted and unscented lotion during the compounding day on hands, arms, and face helps reduce skin shedding. Lotion should be applied after showering and immediately after exiting the compounding area. Applying it before entering can interfere with hand hygiene.

Hand Hygiene and Garbing

USP <797> provides the minimum standard for hand hygiene and garbing. There are many other practical solutions that can be implemented to aid in the minimization of compounding area contamination, especially in the clean room suite. For information specific to HD garbing, see Unit 10.

Before Entering the Sterile Compounding Area

Any individual who will enter must remove any items from their person that are not easily cleanable or are not necessary for compounding. The chapter provides some minimum expectations. Those who enter must[1]:

- Remove personal outer garments – this includes bandanas, coats, hats, sweaters, vests, and scarves.
- Remove all hand, wrist, and other exposed jewelry – this includes any piercings that could interfere with the effectiveness of garbing or otherwise increase the risk of CSP contamination. Any jewelry that cannot be removed must be covered.
- Not wear earbuds or headphones – these are not necessary for compounding and can cause personnel distraction. They are also a significant source of contamination.
- Not bring electronic devices that are not necessary for compounding or other required tasks – this means no cell phones. Cell phones are both a distraction and a contamination risk.
- Wipe eyeglasses, if worn – personal glasses are also a significant contamination risk. Personnel should wipe the frames of their glasses with a one-step bactericidal disinfectant cleaner and the lenses with lens wipes.[10]

Although the above list contains "chapter musts," there is an opportunity to make exceptions. The designated person(s) may permit accommodations provided that the quality of the CSP and environment are not affected.[1] It is critical that any organization that allows for an accommodation thoroughly considers the risks and the precedent it sets for other possible accommodation requests. Any accommodation must be documented by including the date, staff member affected, the accommodation, the length of time the accommodation will be for, and an assessment of the risk.

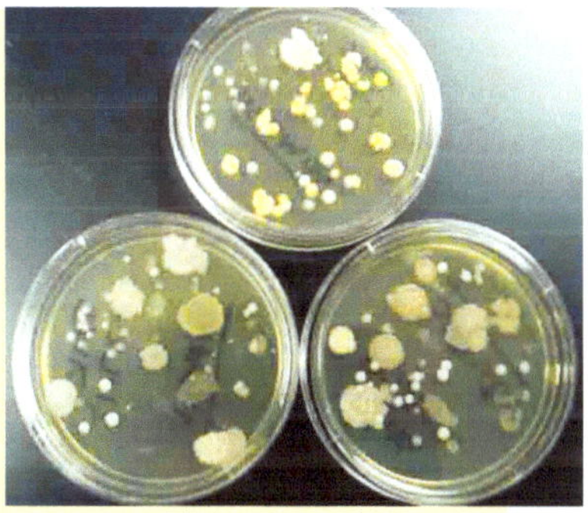
Photo courtesy of Contec, Inc.

Why are cell phones a problem? Cell phones are dirty! One study found that smart phones were contaminated with a median of 15.8 colony forming units (CFU)/cm^2.[11] On a phone that is 15 x 8 cm in size, that equates to roughly 2,370 CFU! In another study that assessed health care workers' phones, *Staphylococcus*, both methicillin-resistant and not, was the most recovered genus, which is expected. However, *Acinetobacter baumannii, Pseudomonas aeruginosa,* and gram-positive spore formers were the next 3 highest recovered. Although lower in the number recovered, *Klebsiella pneumonia* and *Escherichia coli* were also recovered.[12] All of these microorganisms could be pathogenic to a patient if administered via a contaminated CSP.

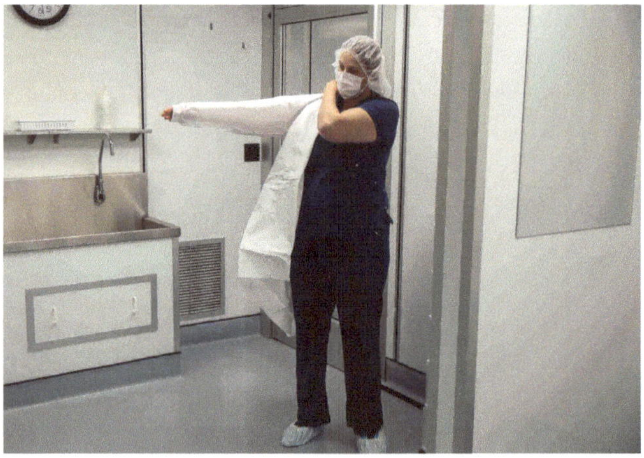

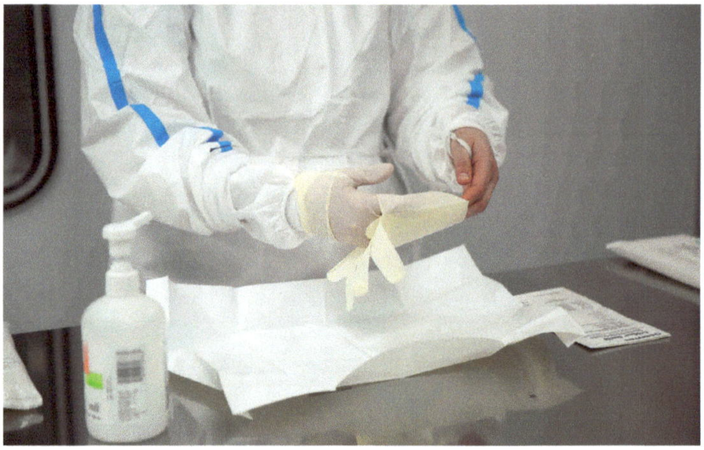

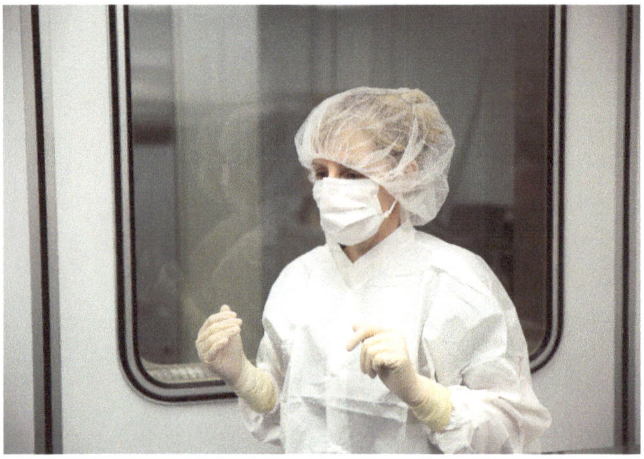

Photos courtesy of Contec, Inc.

Hand Hygiene and Garbing Procedure

Each sterile compounding organization is responsible for defining in its SOPs the hand hygiene and garbing order at their facility. The order is dependent on the facility layout and the location of the sink used for hand hygiene. Additionally, donning and doffing of garb must be done in a way that reduces contamination risk. The organization must consider this when determining the garbing order. There are some additional USP <797> garbing considerations when developing SOPs.[1]

- Any person entering a sterile compounding area must be properly garbed in accordance with the facility's SOPs.
- The manner of garb storage must protect the garb from contamination. Think about an anteroom that has the sink on the clean side of the line of demarcation (LOD). How could gowns be stored to limit contamination risk?
- Skin must not be exposed inside the ISO Class 5 PEC. Gloves must not be donned or doffed inside the PEC.
- Donning and doffing garb ***should not*** occur in the anteroom or the SCA at the same time.

Many home infusion organizations will compound Category 2 CSPs and have the sink on the clean side of the LOD. Let's review the garbing order for this scenario in detail.

1. Tie back hair and wipe glasses outside the anteroom
2. Enter the anteroom and remain on the dirty side of the LOD
3. Don a low-lint facemask, low-lint head cover that covers the hair and ears, and if needed, a low-lint cover for facial hair
    a. The order of donning the facemask and head cover is dependent on the type of mask the facility uses. If the facemasks have loops, they are donned first. If the facemasks tie, the head cover is donned first, and the ties go over the head cover.
    b. Don facial hair covers over the mask. This aids in comfort.

Practical Solution: *Sometimes a head cover and facial hair cover are not sufficient. A hood may be necessary to contain a large beard, a lot of hair, or to cover a religious head covering.*

4. Don low-lint shoe covers one at a time crossing over the LOD

Practical Solution: *Shoes are dirty! To help reduce the microbial contamination from shoes, consider donning dedicated facility shoes that are worn only within the immediate pharmacy area. They are donned before entering the anteroom and are never worn outside the building or into "dirty areas" like patient care areas or warehouses. Donning dedicated shoes does not replace the need for shoe covers.*

5. Wash hands
    a. Clean under fingernails under warm running water using a disposable nail cleaner
    b. Wash hands and forearms up to the elbows with soap and water for at least 30 seconds. Soap must be in a nonrefillable container and brushes must not be used to clean the hands and forearms
    c. Dry hands and forearms up to the elbows completely with low-lint disposable towels or wipers. Hand dryers must not be used

Practical Solution: *Hand washing is one of the activities where personnel cut corners, which is unfortunate because it is a critical part of contamination control. Even though the chapter only requires the use of a nail pick if there is visible dirt, consider using a nail pick every hand washing.*

6. Don a low-lint garment with sleeves that fit snugly around the wrists and an enclosed neck. Gowns are most commonly used; however, a 1-piece coverall is also a common option.

Practical Solution: *Consider something that snaps, or zips closed in the front. Isolation gowns that tie in the back usually do not fully cover the back and can allow for particles from the clothing to be released into the compounding area. Gowns that fully close aid in funneling particles toward the floor, which is particularly helpful in the clean room suite, as this allows the particles to be more quickly removed by the low wall air returns.*

7. Sanitize hands
    a. Apply an alcohol-based hand sanitizer to dry skin following the manufacturer's instructions for the volume of product to use and application procedures
    b. Apply the product to one hand and rub hands together, covering all surfaces of hands and fingers
    c. Allow hands to dry thoroughly before donning sterile gloves
8. Don sterile, powder-free gloves in a classified room

For those sterile compounding organizations that compound Category 3 CSPs, additional garbing requirements must be met, even if Category 3 CSPs are not prepared on a given day.[1]

- There can be no exposed skin in the buffer room. The face and neck must be covered. To accomplish this, a hood and goggles must be worn.
- All low-lint garb must be sterile.
- Disposable garb must not be reused. Laundered garb must not be reused without first being laundered and sterilized. The sterilization cycle must be validated.

What's the harm in donning and doffing garb at the same time? Likely none if the established procedures do not potentially cause risk to the freshly donned garb. What is more of a concern is someone washing hands and splashing water while another person is donning a gown. Be aware of your surroundings when donning garb and discard any garb that may become grossly contaminated.

But the sink is outside of the anteroom! Having a sink outside the anteroom requires a slightly different garbing sequence that incorporates more frequent hand sanitization.

1. Tie back hair and wipe glasses outside the anteroom
2. Wash hands
3. Enter the anteroom and remain on the dirty side of the LOD
4. Sanitize hands
5. Don a low-lint facemask, low-lint head cover that covers the hair and ears, and if needed, a low-lint cover for facial hair
6. Don low-lint shoe covers 1 at a time crossing over the LOD
7. Sanitize hands
8. Don a low-lint garment with sleeves that fit snugly around the wrists and an enclosed neck
9. Sanitize hands
10. Don sterile, powder-free gloves in a classified room

Garb Integrity and Reuse

Have you ever gotten a hole in your glove or a tear in your shoe cover? What did you do?

The integrity of the garb is important. Be sure to check garb for holes and tears during donning and throughout the duration of compounding. Garb must be replaced immediately if it becomes visibly soiled or if its integrity is compromised.[1]

There is some garb that may be reused, under certain conditions. Personnel compounding Category 1 and Category 2 CSPs may reuse a gown during the same shift, as long as it is maintained in a classified area or inside the perimeter of an SCA. When exiting the compounding area, garb, except for gowns, cannot be reused and must be discarded or laundered. Items like goggles and respirators must be disinfected according to facility SOPs.[1]

Material Transfer

Introducing items and equipment into the SEC and PEC is a necessary process for sterile compounding, but it is also a potential avenue for the introduction of microbial contamination. We don't usually think about what we can't see, but 60% of packaging is contaminated with bacteria and 40% with bacterial spores.[13] Each sterile compounding organization must define procedures for moving supplies, components, and drugs in its SOPs.

Transferring to the SEC

The process of introducing items into the sterile compounding area is based on the design of the SEC, but the general principles are the same for all designs.[1]

1. The item must be wiped with the facility-designated agent.
2. The agent must not affect the packaging integrity of the item.
3. The agent can be a sporicidal disinfectant, EPA-registered disinfectant, or sterile 70% IPA.
    a. If a sporicidal disinfectant or EPA-registered disinfectant are used, dwell time must be met.
    b. If sterile 70% IPA is used, it must be allowed to dry.
4. Low-lint wipers must be used.
5. The wiping procedure must not render the product label unreadable.
6. Personnel wiping the items must wear gloves.

Practical Solution: *Although the chapter allows for the use of sterile 70% IPA, it may not be the most effective agent at removing microbial contamination, especially spores. One study indicated that when using sterile 70% IPA for material transfer that only 27.6% of spores would be removed through mechanical wiping.[13] Be sure to evaluate the efficacy of the agent chosen for use during material transfer in the SEC. One way to do this is to review viable surface sampling data. Significant recovery of spore-forming bacteria and mold may indicate poor material transfer practices. If this is the case, switching to a sporicidal disinfectant cleaner for material transfer may be warranted.*

For those with an SCA, items are wiped as they are transferred across the perimeter line, likely going from one cart to another. Those with clean room suites have 2 options for transferring materials: through the anteroom or through pass-through chambers. Even if your facility has pass-through chambers, it is likely that some materials and equipment will be too large and need to be transferred through the anteroom. This transfer is

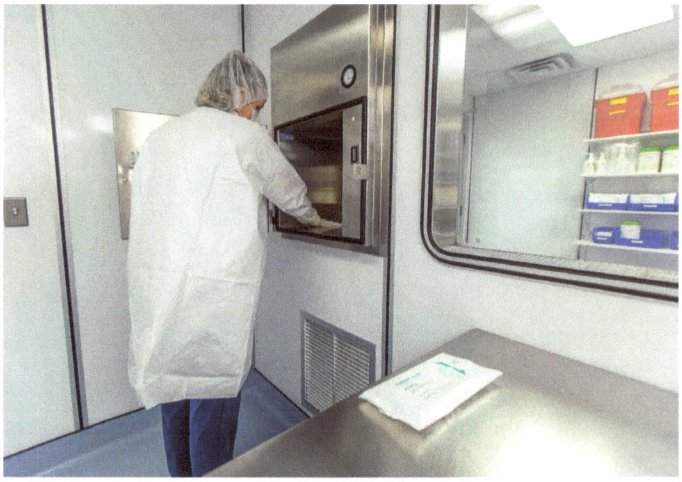

Photo courtesy of Contec, Inc.

best done by bringing the items into the anteroom on a cart, which remains on the dirty side of the LOD. Then the items are wiped as determined by facility SOPs and placed on a clean cart staged on the clean side of the LOD. For those with pass-through chambers from the unclassified space to the classified space, items and equipment are wiped with the designated agent before being transferred into the pass-through chamber. Facilitates should have an area designated for this purpose which is kept it clean and uncluttered.

Practical Solution: *During a high-volume material transfer through the anteroom, which will take significant time, consider having the individual performing the transfer be fully garbed. This will help maintain the cleanliness of the anteroom, especially if it is ISO Class 7.*

Transferring Into the PEC

A critical part of aseptic technique is the transfer of items into the PEC. USP <797> provides guidance on transferring items into the PEC.[1]

1. Wipe with sterile 70% IPA.
2. Use sterile low-lint wipers.
3. Allow to dry before use.
4. The wiping procedure must not render the product label unreadable.

Many of the supplies used in sterile compounding are received in sealed containers designed to keep them sterile until opening. The sterile items may be removed from the covering as the supplies are introduced into the PEC without the need to wipe the individual sterile supply items with sterile 70% IPA.[1]

Transferring materials into the sterile compounding area is a mundane process. Because this is a critical part of contamination control, personnel need to be taught not only what to do and how to do it, but why the proper transfer of materials is so important. And remember, material transfer is a 2-step process.

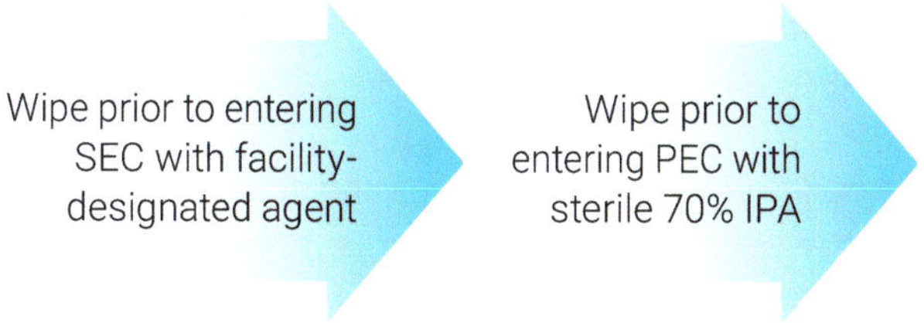

Wipe prior to entering SEC with facility-designated agent
Wipe prior to entering PEC with sterile 70% IPA

Aseptic Technique and SEC Behavior

As mentioned previously, USP <797> mentions aseptic technique, but provides very few specifics. This leaves the sterile compounding organization with the responsibility of defining the behaviors and processes associated with ensuring sterility of the CSP. When developing the necessary SOPs, there are 6 general categories associated with aseptic technique and SEC behavior that should be considered:

1. Movement and behavior
2. Organization
3. Comfort
4. Communication
5. Concentration
6. Sanitization

Movement and Behavior

Sterile compounding personnel need to move slowly and deliberately through the sterile compounding area and when working in the PEC. This reduces the number of particles generated. Exhibit 1 provides a visual of just how many particles compounding personal can generate.

Observing the behavior of sterile compounding personnel provides insight into the true aseptic technique of an individual. Essentially everything that individual does in the sterile compounding area defines their ability to properly maintain the sterile compounding environment and produce safe medications. Proper use of first air is the most critical behavior in ensuring the sterility of a preparation.

Have you heard the term first air before? What does it mean to you?

USP <797> defines first air as *"the air exiting the HEPA filter in a unidirectional air stream."*[1] This definition lacks the clarification that the air exiting the HEPA filter must not touch anything else before it reaches the critical sites of vials, bags, needles, etc. If the air touches anything before touching the critical site, it may have picked up contaminating particles. Proper hand positioning during aseptic manipulations and a properly organized work surface in the PEC help ensure first air reaches the critical sites.

Which airflow direction do you work in when compounding sterile preparations? How does the airflow

Exhibit 1

Skin Particles Generated Based on Different Movements[14]

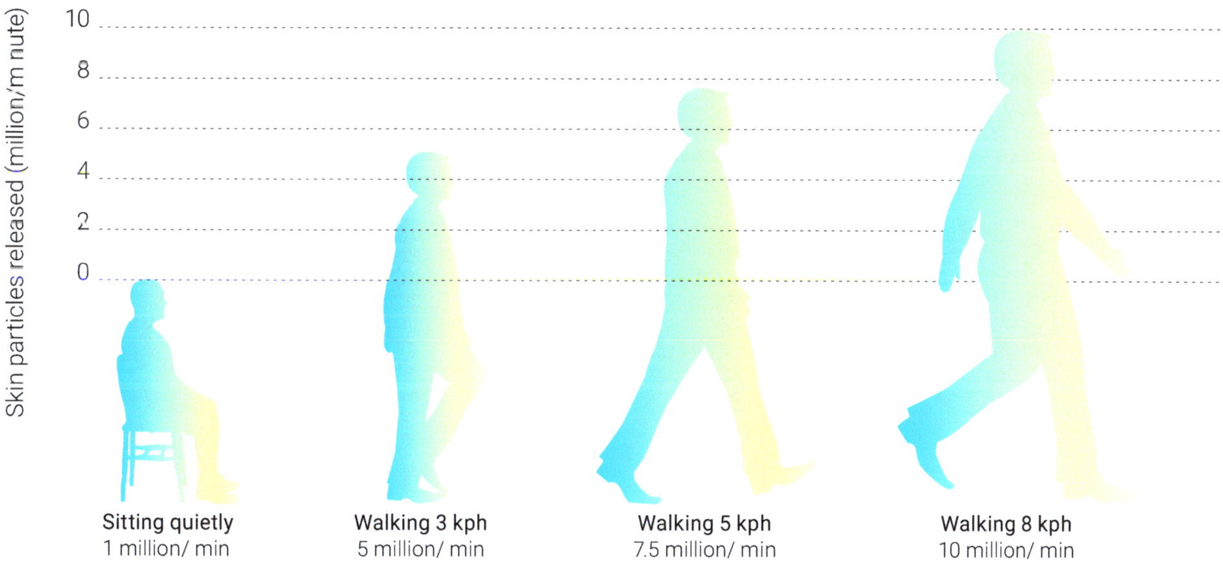

Exhibit 2
PEC Airflow Direction Comparison

Horizontal Flow	Vertical Flow
Air moves from the back of the PEC to the opening	Air moves from the top of the PEC to the work surface
Device: LAFWs	Device: LAFWs, BSCs, CAIs, CACIs
Non-hazardous compounding	Non-hazardous (LAFWs only) and hazardous compounding
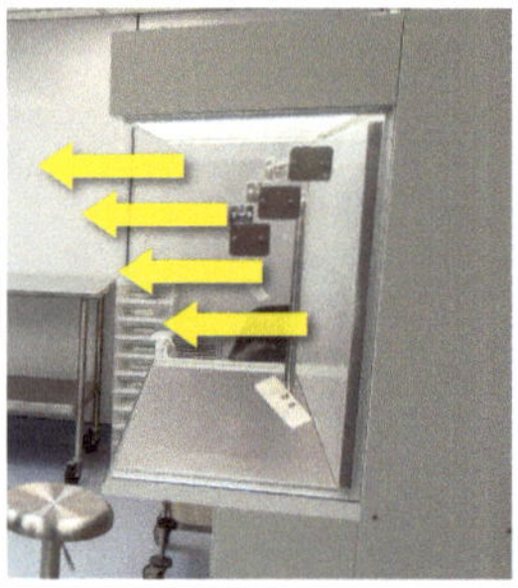	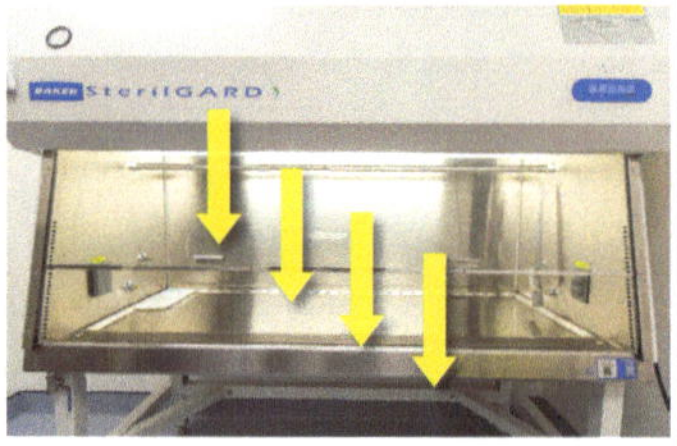

affect your compounding technique and behavior? Exhibit 2 describes the 2 different types of airflow that you may work in.

Practical Solution: *When training sterile compounding personnel about first air, consider using a smoke source as a learning tool. Smoke testing provides staff the opportunity to "see" the airflow. During the training, use the smoke to evaluate the airflow during different compounding procedures, specifically looking at:*

- *Proper hand positioning for the airflow direction*
- *Vial and bag positioning*
- *Working under the IV bar in vertical flow*
- *Working behind items in horizontal flow*
- *How automated compounding devices can significantly affect airflow in the DCA*

In addition to proper use of first air, other good compounding behaviors include but are not limited to:

- Use of sterile instruments when touching sterile sites
- Arms and elbows off the work surface
- Head does not enter PEC
- Not touching and/or blocking critical sites, including the plunger of a syringe
- Working in the DCA
- Proper compounding pressure technique
- Garbing changes when needed
- Visual verification – no syringe pullback
- Limitation of aseptic breaks
- Leaving dropped items on the floor until an appropriate time to retrieve them

Organization

How do you organize your compounding workflow? What does the work surface of the PEC look like? Why do you place the items where you do?

Sterile compounding organizations should design a workflow to limit movement in and out of the compounding area and the PEC. This reduces the microbial contamination risk and makes the compounding process more efficient. The best way to identify proper workflow is to observe current practices and talk with staff about improvements. Good organization ultimately reduces particles and microbial contamination.
Staff may have preferences in how they organize the PEC work surface; however, the workflow should be unidirectional. Either left to right or right to left. The example below is working from left to right.

Staged items → DCA → Trash

It is also important that when working in the horizontal flow PEC that items are placed side by side instead of front to back, as this could block first air from reaching critical sites.

PEC work surface organization is also defined by airflow smoke pattern testing and equipment used in the compounding process. Large pieces of equipment like a PN compounder or a workflow management system block air exiting the HEPA filter. Once that air touches the equipment it is no longer first air, and it must find a way to exit the PEC. It could roll over the top or around the

Don't Have a Workflow Management System? The Institute for Safe Medication Practices (ISMP) states that if a workflow management system is not used, multiple CSPs for one or multiple patients can only be done at the same time if they are the same drug, same dose, and same administration route.[18] This form of line clearance is a critical component of patient safety.

sides. If during the smoke pattern test it shows that this air enters what was thought to be the DCA, the location of the DCA must be adjusted. Sharing a video of this testing provides staff with a visual of where they can make aseptic connections.

Line clearance is a manufacturing concept, mentioned in the Code of Federal Regulations, that can be applied to sterile compounding. The idea is to prevent "mix-ups and cross-contamination by physical or spatial separation from operations on other drug products."[17] When applied to sterile compounding, it ensures that vials, CSPs, labels, etc. from a previous patient are removed before starting the preparation for the next patient.

Comfort

USP <797> indicates that the compounding area must be designed to be a comfortable working environment. Temperature and humidity are important in ensuring this requirement. Remember, the suggested clean room suite maximum temperature is 20° C/68° F and maximum is humidity 60%. Be sure to consider the comfort of staff when fully garbed.

Properly fitting garb also contributes to comfort and limits microbial contamination risk. Gowns need to be sized to allow mobility but should not be so big as to result in not being fully closed at the neck. Properly fitted facemasks may also be a problem. When facemasks don't fit properly, staff tend to touch the mask to adjust. Anytime a garb adjustment is made, consideration should be given to changing gloves before resuming work.

Sterile compounding consists of a variety of repetitive movements. The ergonomics of compounding techniques need to be considered to keep staff free from injury. Uncomfortable movements may result in staff making inappropriate adjustments that could compromise aseptic technique. There are 10 principles of ergonomics that need to be considered.[15]

1. Working in neutral posture
2. Reducing excessive force
3. Keeping everything within easy reach
4. Working at the proper height
5. Reducing excessive motions
6. Minimizing fatigue and static load
7. Minimizing pressure points
8. Providing clearance
9. Moving, exercising, and stretching
10. Maintaining comfortable environment

Ergonomics: What to Look for[16]

- Neutral posture back, head and neck, elbows, wrists
- Chairs or stools at work-surface height
- Excessive force activities
- "Reach envelope" – the area that can be reached without stretching
- Repetitive movements

If any actions could result in injury or shortcuts, the action should be evaluated for possible alternative options.

Communication

Communication in the compounding area is essential to operations but can also be a contamination risk. USP <797> does not address avenues for communication, so it is important for the organization to define how those working within the compounding area will communicate with those outside and what the expectations are for communication within the compounding area. Unnecessary talking can be a distraction and talking in the PEC can be a contamination risk. A communication system is an important tool for compounding efficiency. When evaluating communication systems, consider cleanability, ease of use, and accessibility.

Concentration

Preparing a CSP is a complex task that requires focus to ensure safety. This should be openly discussed during initial and ongoing training of sterile compounding personnel. Conversations while preparing a CSP should be limited to compounding and the task at hand. Staff should also turn away from the PEC to speak, so they are not talking directing into the device. Cell phones can be distracting and a significant contamination risk. Based on USP <797>, "*only furniture, equipment, and other materials necessary for performing compounding activities are permitted in a classified area or SCA....*"[2] This means no cell phones, unless they are essential to the work performed. However, if they are essential to compounding activities, like video recording a smoke study, there must be specific policies regarding how to properly transfer the phone into the sterile compounding environment.

Practical Solution: *Many like to listen to music while working. For some it can help concentration, while it may be a distraction for others, as music preferences can affect concentration. If the facility allows it, here are some tips.*[19]

- Keep the volume low
- Avoid music with lyrics
- Choose slow, instrumental music
- Choose commercial-free music

Sanitization

Sterile compounding personnel use sterile 70% IPA to sanitize many different surfaces over the course of a workday and sanitization occurs more frequently than disinfection. These surfaces include gloves, components, supplies, critical sites, the PEC work surface, and frequently touched surfaces. During compounding, gloves are sanitized after staff touch non-sterile surfaces (screens, chairs, etc.), before gloved hands enter the PEC, immediately prior to performing any aseptic procedures, and at any point they may be contaminated. Components and supplies are sanitized when transferred into the PEC. Critical sites are sanitized during the compounding process. It is important to also sanitize frequently touched surfaces during the compounding day. Items like tables, carts, pass-throughs, and workflow systems can harbor microorganisms and frequent sanitization lowers the bioburden on these surfaces.

Summary

The success of a sterile compounding organization hinges on the aseptic technique of its personnel. Low-linting garbing materials, proper cleaning and disinfecting procedures, and well-designed facilities cannot make up for poor behavior and technique. USP <797> provides basic guidance and leaves it to the sterile compounding organization to define exactly what aseptic technique looks like to them. SOPs should address garbing, material transfer, clean room behavior, and compounding technique.

References

1. United States Pharmacopeia. <797> Pharmaceutical Compounding—Sterile Preparations. Revision. November 2022.
2. Kastango ES. Spread the Word: Aseptic Technique Prevents Infection. Pharmacy Purchasing and Products Magazine. April 2009.
3. Personal Hygiene. Encyclopedia.com. 2019. Accessed June 11, 2022.
4. Berg RD. The indigenous gastrointestinal microflora. *Trends Microbiol.* 1996;4:430–5.
5. Milstone LM. "Epidermal Desquamation." *Journal of Dermatological Science* 36, no. 3 (December 1, 2004): 131–40.
6. Hospodsky D, Qian J, Nazaroff WW, et al. Human occupancy as a source of indoor airborne bacteria. *PLoS One.* 2012;7(4):e34867. doi:10.1371/journal.pone.0034867
7. Centers for Disease Control and Prevention. Keeping Hands Clean. Water, Sanitation & Environmentally-related Hygiene. Last reviewed December 4, 2019.
8. Goldstein K. Cosmetics in clean rooms ... again? *Solid State Technology.* 2001.
9. U.S. Food and Drug Administration (FDA). Is It a Cosmetic, a Drug, or Both? (Or Is It Soap?). August 24, 2020.
10. CriticalPoint. Pearls of Knowledge. Best Practices for Garbing for Nonhazardous Sterile Compounding Areas. May 2019.
11. Kõljalg S, Mändar R, Sõber T, Rööp T, Mändar R. High level bacterial contamination of secondary school students' mobile phones. *Germs.* 2017 Jun 1;7(2):73-77. doi: 10.18683/germs.2017.1111. PMID: 28626737; PMCID: PMC5466825.
12. Morubagal RR, Shivappa SG, Mahale RP, Neelambike SM. Study of bacterial flora associated with mobile phones of healthcare workers and non-healthcare workers. *Iran J Microbiol.* 2017 Jun;9(3):143-151. PMID: 29225753; PMCID: PMC5719508.
13. Cockcroft MG, Hepworth D, Rhodes JC, Addison P. Validation of liquid transfer disinfection techniques for transfer of components into hospital pharmacy clean room. *Hospital Pharmacist.* January 2001, 8(8):226-232.
14. Particle Measuring Systems. Beginner Guide to Particle Technology. Retrieved May 31, 2022.
15. Wagle K. Ergonomics and its 10 principles. Public Health Notes. August 25, 2018. *Ergonomics for trainers.* University of Massachusetts Lowell, Train-the-Trainer Program.
16. Tribble D. Ergonomics of Sterile Compounding. ASHP Midyear Clinical Meeting and Exhibition. 2021.
17. Code of Federal Regulations. Title 21. Chapter I. Subpart G. § 211.130 Packaging and labeling operations.
18. Institute for Safe Medication Practices. ISMP Guidelines for Sterile Compounding and the Safe Use of Sterile Compounding Technology. 2022.
19. Raypole C. Music and Studying: It's Complicated. Healthline.com. July 29, 2020.

Summary: Hand Hygiene and Garbing

Before Reporting to Work

- Make sure you are healthy enough to enter
- Moisturize skin and keep short, natural nails
- Shower daily, preferably in the morning
- Remove all cosmetics

Before Entering the Compounding Area

- Wear laundered clothing
- Remove ear buds
- Don dedicated shoes
- Finish food and drink
- Tie back hair
- Follow policy for badges
- Remove all visible jewelry
- Wipe glasses

Garbing Order Based on Sink Location

Clean Side of LOD	Dirty Side of LOD	Outside Anteroom
1. Secure hair, clean glasses 2. Enter anteroom, don face and head covers 3. Don shoe covers 4. Perform hand hygiene 5. Don gown 6. Apply hand rub 7. Don sterile gloves	1. Secure hair, clean glasses 2. Enter anteroom, don face and head covers 3. Perform hand hygiene 4. Don shoe covers 5. Apply hand rub 6. Don gown 7. Apply hand rub 8. Don sterile gloves	1. Secure hair, clean glasses 2. Perform hand hygiene 3. Enter anteroom 4. Apply hand rub 5. Don face and head covers 6. Don shoe covers 7. Apply hand rub 8. Don gown 9. Apply hand rub 10. Don sterile gloves

UNIT 5
Summary: Hand Hygiene and Garbing

Aseptic Practices

During material transfer, look for:

- Use of facility-designated agent and low-linting wipers
- Wiping and not just spraying
- Dwell time
- Label integrity

When evaluating aseptic behavior, look for:

- Slow and controlled movement
- Proper hand position for the airflow direction
- Vial and bag positioning
- Use of sterile instruments when touching sterile sites
- Arms and elbows off the work surface
- Head does not enter the PEC
- Not touching critical sites, including the syringe plunger
- Working in the DCA
- Proper compounding pressure technique

UNIT 6

Viable Air and Surface Sampling

Microorganisms are everywhere. Even in the sterile compounding environment. To understand the risk that microorganisms pose to the final CSP, it is necessary to collect viable air and surface samples. Sample collection provides a semi-quantitative snapshot in time of the number and types of bacteria, yeast, and mold that were in the sterile compounding area during that specific collection. This data allows sterile compounding organizations to make informed decisions regarding changes to workflow and procedures, resulting in process improvement. In this unit, we will discuss some of the benefits and limitations of viable sampling, as well as the requirements and practical solutions that ensure a successful sampling program.

Viable Sampling Benefits and Limitations

USP General Chapter <797> requires the collection of viable air and surface sampling. Through this sampling, the sterile compounding organization can understand the environmental quality of the compounding area. And through the development of a robust viable sampling program, it will allow for the identification of potential contamination risks, trending of data, and implementation of corrective actions in the event of exceeded action levels.

The purpose of the viable sampling program *"is to confirm that the conditions in the clean room are consistent and appropriate. By performing routine sampling, a monitoring program can identify changes in the recovery of microorganisms, which in turn can identify possible changes in the state of control of the clean room."*[1] However, viable sampling comes with its limitations. And it is critical that those responsible for the viable sampling plan recognize them.

Limitation #1

The designated person should review viable sampling results frequently to ensure a state of control, but monitoring can neither prove nor disprove sterility of the CSP.[2] Viable sampling must not be used solely as a release test for compounded sterile preparations.

Limitation #2

Viable sampling cannot and need not identify and quantify all microorganisms in the sterile compounding area.[2] Quantitative sampling is impossible–there would be no way to sample all the air and all the surfaces in a clean room. So, viable sampling is semi-quantitative.[1] This is a significant limitation, and it exists in part because of the growth-based methods used in sample

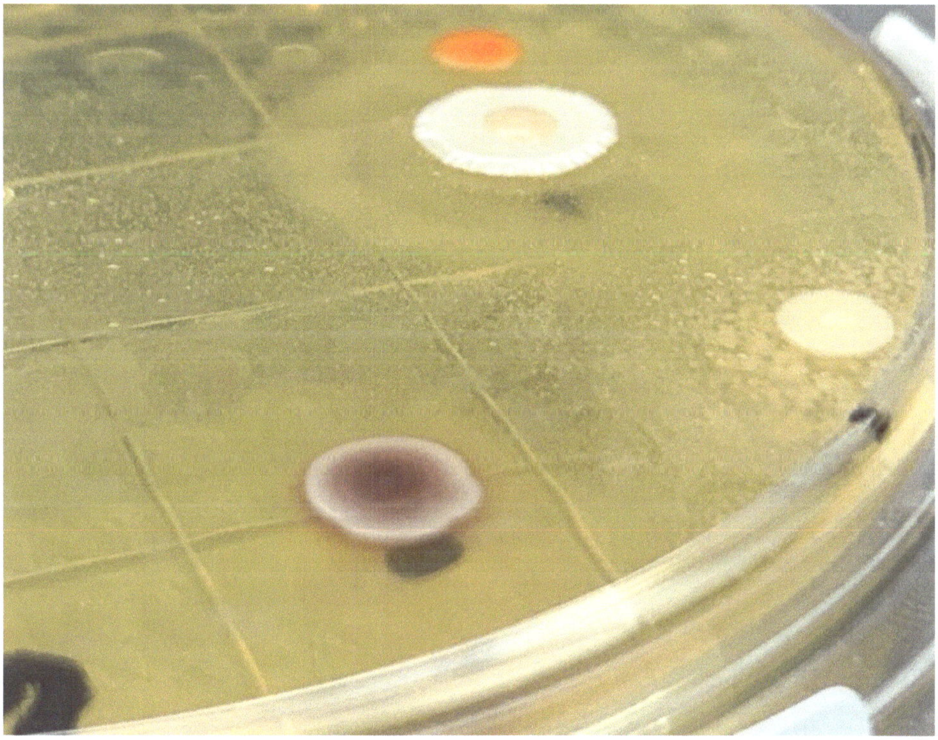

Photo courtesy of Pure Microbiology, LLC

Are you getting all zeros on your viable sampling report? This might not be a good thing. We expect to find microorganisms in the buffer and anterooms, especially during the workday. If you are consistently not recovering any growth during dynamic operating conditions, this is a concern. First, confirm that cleaning is not occurring immediately before sampling. Cleaning prior to sampling defeats the purpose. A viable sampling program is intended to recover the microorganisms that are present, evaluate the results, and take appropriate corrective actions which leads to process improvement. Second, be sure samples are collected during dynamic operating conditions, which is a USP <797> requirement. Staff must be working, and the collection should be performed toward the end of the shift or compounding day to represent worst-case conditions. Third, the media could have been compromised and is no longer able to support growth. Consider having growth promotion testing performed on the media by a contract microbiology laboratory.

collection. Only the microorganisms that proliferate under the conditions presented by the media, incubation time, and incubation temperatures provided will be recovered. Remember that viable sampling is a snapshot of what was happening during collection.[3]

Limitation #3

The sampling plan cannot prove absence of microorganisms, even when no microorganisms are recovered.[2] Microorganisms could still have been present during sampling, they just were not recovered.

The Viable Sampling Program

USP <797> requires the development of a written sampling program. High-level requirements include:[4]

1. Documentation of monitoring procedures, the test results, and the corrective actions
2. Maintenance of all associated records
3. Review of data collected in response to corrective actions to verify the actions taken were effective
4. Collection of impaction air samples and surface samples
5. Analysis of data to detect trends

The sampling program must also include a diagram of the sampling locations, procedures for collecting samples, frequency of sampling, size of samples, time of day of sampling in relation to activities in the compounding area, and action levels.[4] Let's look at each of these requirements in more detail.

Diagram of Sampling Locations

Part of the sampling program is a sampling plan. This plan identifies the locations for viable air and surface collection. The chapter requires a diagram, like the one shown in Exhibit 1. In addition, consider having a list that describes each specific sample location. For example, for S6 in Exhibit 1, the description would read: S6 – Left side of the table. This ensures sampling consistency, regardless of who does the sample collection.

Procedures for Collection Samples

Traditionally, sterile compounding organizations relied on the SOPs of the sampling vendors to describe sampling procedures. With this chapter requirement, facility SOPs must include the "how to" information on sample collection. Even if the facility uses a vendor to collect samples, the expectation is that they follow the facility's SOPs. SOPs need to address:

- **Preparing to Sample**
  - Gathering of materials and media
  - When sampling can occur
  - Transfer of materials into the compounding environment
  - Garbing

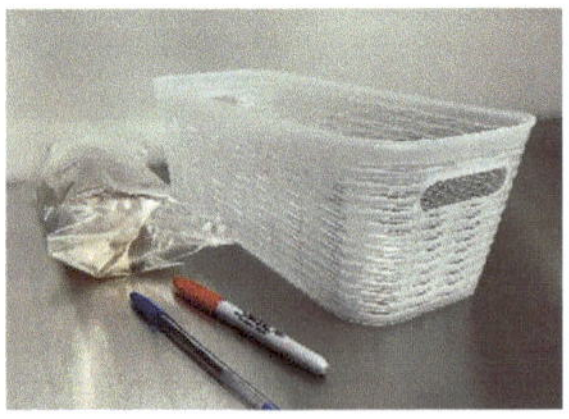

- **Sampling Process**
  - Identification of a work area
  - Sampling order
  - Sampling technique
  - Labeling
  - Documentation

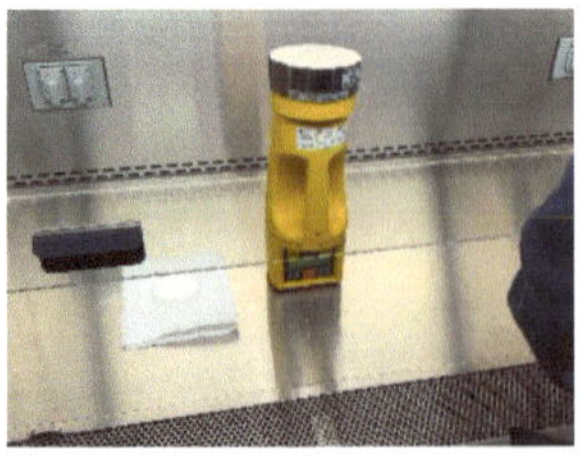

Photos courtesy of Pure Microbiology, LLC

Exhibit 1

Viable Air and Surface Sampling Plan Diagram

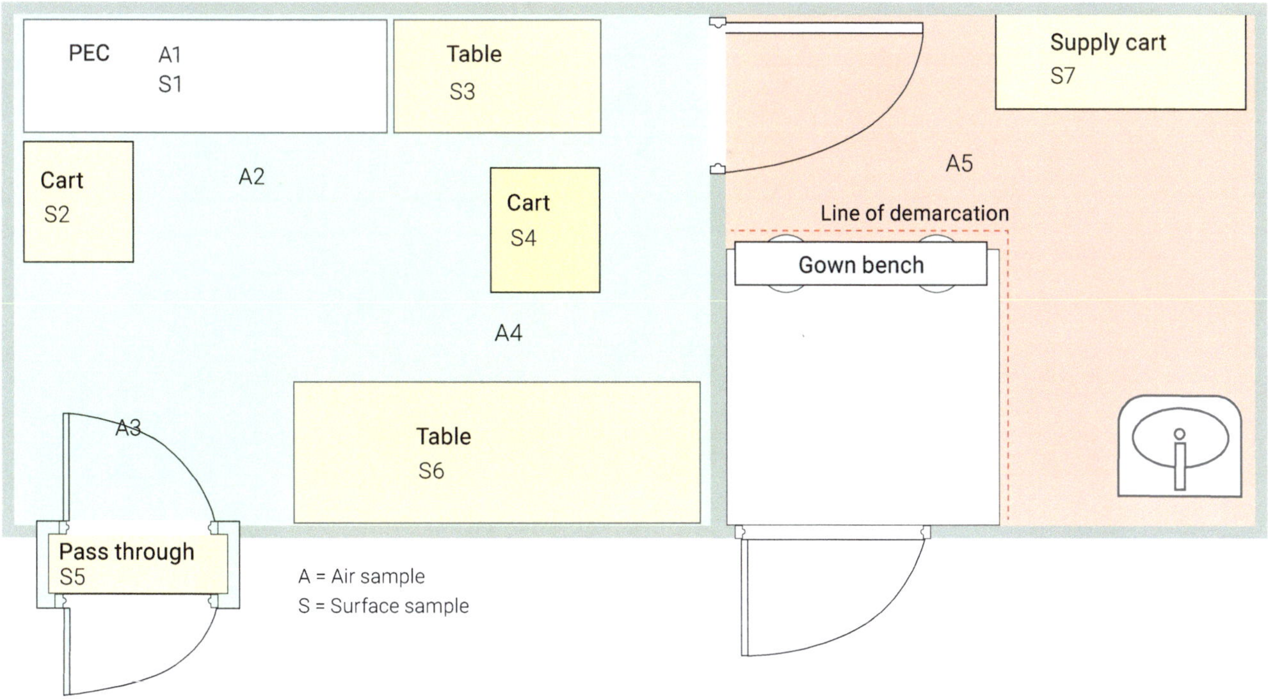

The selection of sample locations will be discussed later in this unit.

- **Completion of Sampling**
  - Verification that all samples were collected
  - Completion of documentation
  - Completion of chain of custody if samples are sent to a laboratory
  - Incubation parameters
  - Shipping of samples if they are sent to a laboratory

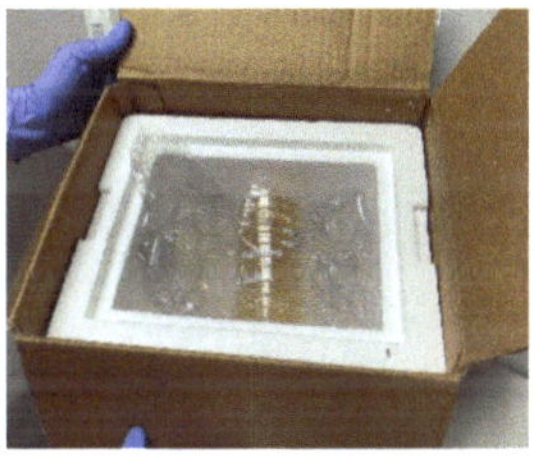

Be sure to share the SOPs with the sampling vendor! A best practice is to share the SOPs with the sampling vendor prior to the vendor's visit. Allow time to schedule a meeting with the vendor to discuss the plan so all parties have a clear understanding of what expectations are.

Frequency of Sampling

USP <797> specifies the frequency of viable air and surface sample collection. These frequencies are based on the categories of CSPs compounded by the sterile compounding organization. Surface sampling is also performed in conjunction with the media fill test. Exhibit 2 describes the required frequencies.

Practical Solution: *USP <797> requires the facility to trend data in order to identify the loss of a microbial state of control. Requirements for Categories 1 and 2 are for air sampling only every 6 months,*

Exhibit 2

Minimum Required Viable Sampling Frequencies[4]

Category	Viable Air	Viable Surface
1 and 2	At least every 6 months	At least monthly
3	• Completed within 30 days prior to the start of any Category 3 compounding • At least monthly regardless of the frequency of compounding Category 3 CSPs	• Completed prior to assigning a BUD longer than USP <797> limits • At least weekly regardless of the frequency of compounding Category 3 CSPs • Conducted within the PEC used to prepare Category 3 CSPs, at the end of each batch before cleaning and disinfection occurs

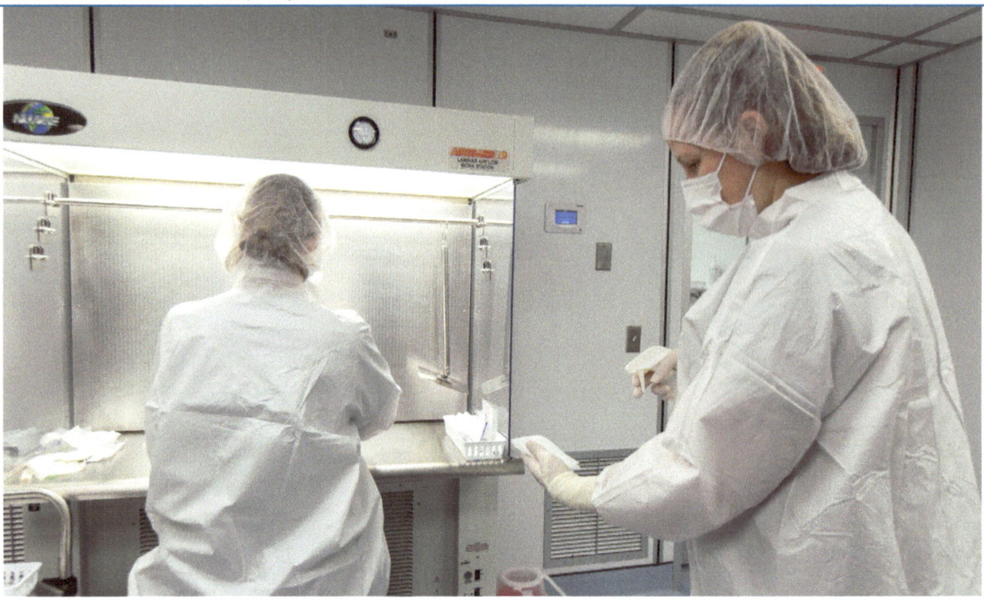

Photo courtesy of Pure Microbiology, LLC

leading to a lack of information for trending. To have a better understanding of the facility, consider collecting viable air samples monthly. This can be completed by a sampling vendor or by organization staff with a purchased air sampler. In addition to the sampling frequencies mentioned, viable sampling is required to be performed:[4]

- *In conjunction with the certification of new facilities and equipment*
- *After any servicing of facilities or equipment*
- *In response to identified problems*
- *In response to identified trends*
- *In response to changes that could impact the sterile compounding environment*

SOPs must address these situations and any others identified by the sterile compounding organization that could require viable sampling.

Size of Samples

Viable air sample collection is done in liters (L). USP <797> requires that 1,000 L of air is collected for each air sample. This is because the viable air sample results are reported in cubic meters (m^3) and there are 1,000 L of air in a cubic meter. This eliminates the need for a calculation when determining the number of colony forming units (CFUs) recovered. Viable surface samples are collected using various collection devices, such as plates, paddles, or slides. The size of the sample collected is based on the device chosen and the results are reported as CFU/sampling device. Contact plates are the recommended sampling device and they are approximated 25 cm^2 in size.

Time of Day of Sampling in Relation to Activities in the Compounding Area

USP <797> specifies that viable air and surface samples must be collected under dynamic operating conditions and that surface samples should be collected *"at the end of a compounding activity or shift but before the area has been cleaned and disinfected."*[4] The sampling program must describe these requirements and the paperwork used to document the sampling session should capture this information.[5] However, viable air and surface sampling under static conditions can supply a baseline of the microorganisms that reside in the facility. Additionally, surface sampling under static conditions after cleaning provides data on cleaning efficacy.

Action Levels

USP <797> provides action levels for both viable air and surface samples, based on the ISO class in which they were sampled. The sterile compounding organization can use the action levels provided by the chapter or institute its own action levels, as long as they are stricter than what is provided by the chapter. Exhibit 3 displays the action levels for both viable air and surface samples under dynamic conditions.

Exhibit 3
USP <797> Prescribed Action Levels for Viable Air and SurfaceSamples[4]

ISO Class	Air Action Level CFU/m^3	Surface Action Level CFU/plate
5	>1	>3
7	>10	>5
8	>100	>50

Choosing Sample Locations

Think about your sampling plan. Do you know how and why sample locations were chosen? Do these locations provide insight to the risk to the CSP?

The selection of viable sampling locations is not an arbitrary act. Locations must be carefully chosen to provide valuable data about CSP contamination risk and the overall state of microbial control. Initially, locations are determined as part of the clean room startup or commissioning. At the time of initial startup, a prospective risk analysis should be conducted with the input from a team of members who understand the compounding process and workflow, engineering controls, and contamination control. This assessment will identify locations, where if microorganisms are found, may result in risk to the final CSP. As part of the assessment, the team should develop a rationale for the sampling locations.

There is no right or wrong to the number of samples collected, however, at a minimum USP <797> requires that each ISO classified environment be sampled. The number of samples chosen needs to strike a balance. Over-sampling can be a contamination risk to the environment, but under-sampling may not provide enough information about the environment. Careful consideration of risk and reduction of contamination sources should guide the sampling intensity.

When choosing locations consider the following:

- Areas at greatest risk of contamination
- High-touch areas that could result in CSP contamination, like workflow systems
- Human activity during compounding
- Entry points from areas of lower classification to those of higher classification
- Areas within and around doors and pass-through chambers
- Location of equipment

The best way to choose locations is to watch work practices. This offers amazing insight into how people move through the space, what they touch, and where components and supplies are staged before they enter the PEC. Exhibit 4 describes sampling locations that should be considered as part of the sampling plan.

Practical Solution: *As was mentioned, samples must be collected in each ISO classified environment. If you have an SCA, the chapter does not require sample collection in*

Exhibit 4

Recommended Viable Air and Surface Locations Based on ISO Classification

ISO Class	Viable Air Samples	Surface Samples
5	• 1 sample in the DCA • If the PEC has more than 1 DCA, both must be sampled • DCA of the main chamber of a RABS • Transfer chamber of a RABS (if it is HEPA purged and classified as class 5)	• 1 sample in the DCA* • DCA of the main chamber of a RABS • Transfer chamber of a RABS • Equipment housed in the PEC
7	• Directly outside the PEC where the staff are located • By workstations • Any area that has higher particle counts • By the pass through chamber door	• Many options, some provide better data on the state of control than others • Staging or work areas near the PEC carts and tables • Interior of the pass-through chamber* • Refrigerators • Shelving • Workflow systems
8	• On the clean side of the line of demarcation • By workstations • Any area that has higher particle counts • By the pass-through chamber door if there is a pass-through to the unclassified space	

* USP <797> required sample location
DCA – direct compounding area
PEC – primary engineering control
RABS – restricted access barrier system

USP <797> recommends the sampling of "frequently touched areas." This language is challenging because there are a lot of frequently touched areas in the clean room suite, but it will not be possible, nor is it necessary, to collect samples on all of them. This is where the risk assessment comes in. Identify the frequently touched areas and evaluate each to determine if the location is truly a risk to the final CSP. For example, contamination on a staging cart next to a PEC used by a technician compounding PN would be a great place for a sample location, while the door handle on the door between the anteroom and the unclassified space doesn't provide any valuable data.

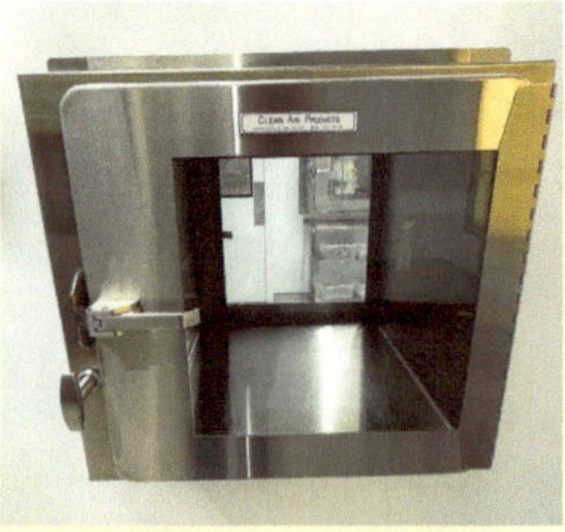

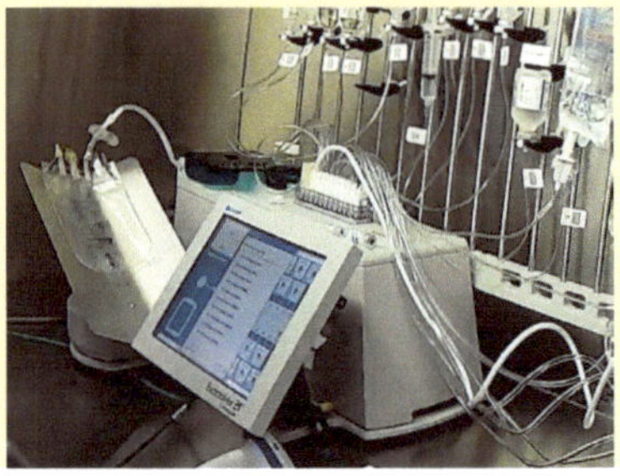

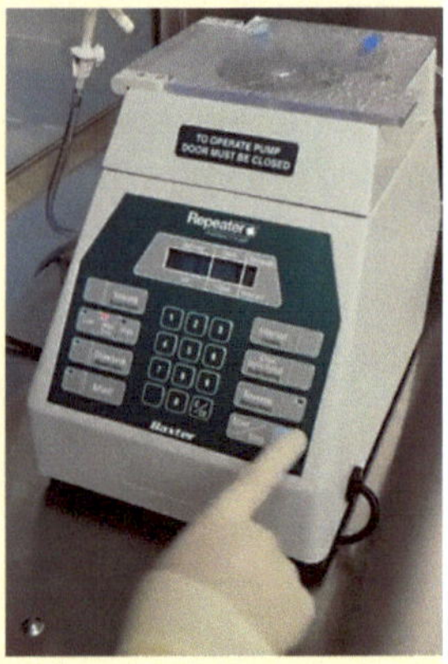

Photos courtesy of Optum

the room, as it is not ISO classified. However, collecting 1 air and 1 surface sample within the perimeter of the SCA can be beneficial in an investigation in the event there is an exceeded action level in the PEC. These samples do not have action levels and are for information purposes only.

Media Selection

Trypticase soy agar (TSA) is required for both viable and surface sample collection. This general growth medium will support the growth of bacteria, yeast, and mold. Facilities can also use a fungal medium, such as malt extract agar (MEA) or sabouraud dextrose agar (SDA), in conjunction with TSA. If this is done, both types of media are used to sample at each designated sample location. For the collection of surface samples, the media must contain neutralizers, such as lecithin and polysorbate 80.[4] These neutralizers are added to the media to neutralize any cleaning agent residues that could be left on the surface, causing possible false negative results.

Ordering media can be confusing. There are so many variations of TSA plates. When ordering media, be sure to verify:

1. The type of plate. TSA is available in contact plates and settle plates. Choose the proper type based on your sampling needs.

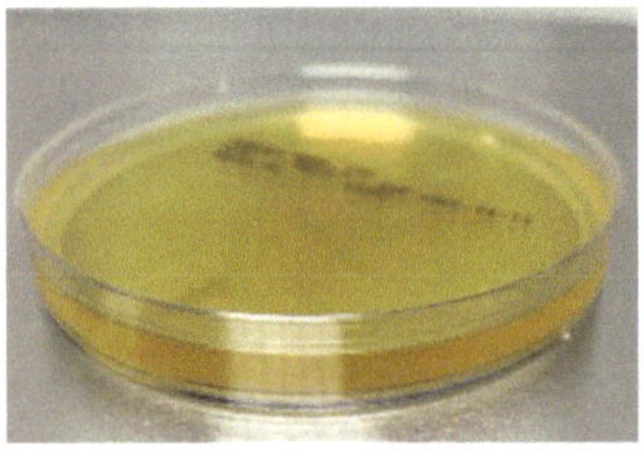

Settle plate

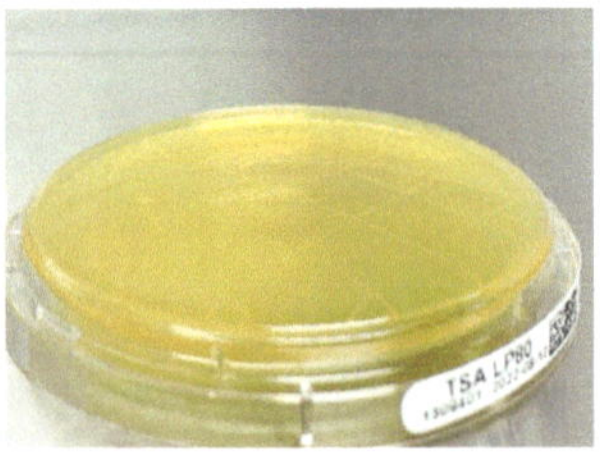

Contact plate

2. That the contact plates (or other sampling devices) have lecithin and polysorbate 80 (also known as Tween 80)
3. That the media is irradiated and at least double bagged.
4. That the storage conditions are conducive to your facility. Some can be stored at room temperature while other media needs to be refrigerated and this can vary depending on the type of plate and the manufacturer. Be sure to have adequate space to accommodate the storage of your purchase.
5. The expiration date. Media has a relatively short shelf-life, which makes it challenging to order enough to cover the sampling needs for the year. Some manufacturers will provide the expiration date of stock if you contact them.

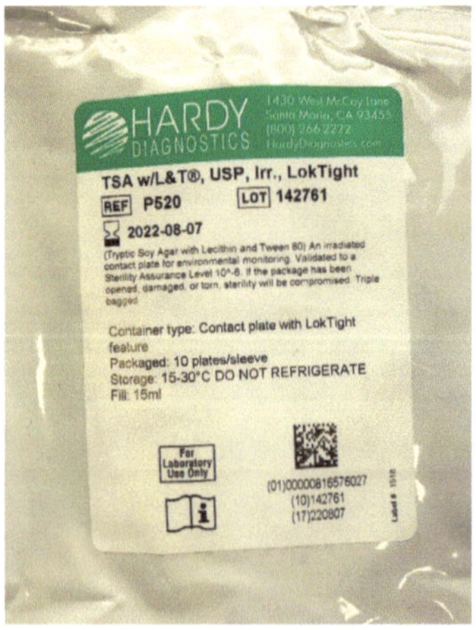

Photos courtesy of Pure Microbiology, LLC

A label on packaged sampling plates. Note that the media is:

1. TSA with lecithin and tween 80
2. Irradiated
3. To be stored at room temperature
4. Labeled with the expiration date.

Practical Solution: *Terminally sterilized versus aseptically filled media – Sterile media is prepared in 2 ways: terminally sterilized and aseptically filled. Keeping in mind sterility assurance concepts, an aseptically filled product results in the probability that 1 item out of 1,000 will be contaminated, while a terminally sterilized product results in the probability that 1 item out of 1,000,000 will be contaminated. Yes, they both result in a sterile product, but the terminally sterilized product provides much better assurance of this. When it comes to viable sampling, it makes sound scientific sense to start with terminally sterilized media, which is accomplished through gamma irradiation.*

Upon receipt of the media, review the certificate of analysis (COA) to ensure the media meets the expected growth promotion, pH, and sterility requirements. Retain the COA in the event the media is recalled in the future, or you have an issue with the media.

Viable Air Sampling

A volumetric, impaction air sampler is used to collect viable air samples. With this technology, the air sampler is programmed to collect a predetermined amount of air, which impacts the surface of the agar plate, capturing any microorganisms present. This collection method is also known as active air sampling. In contrast, the use of settling plates to collect microorganisms that fall out of the air, is known as passive air sampling. USP <797> requires active air sampling and that the air sampling device be calibrated and maintained as required by the manufacturer. Sample collection is performed according to the manufacturer's instructions for use.

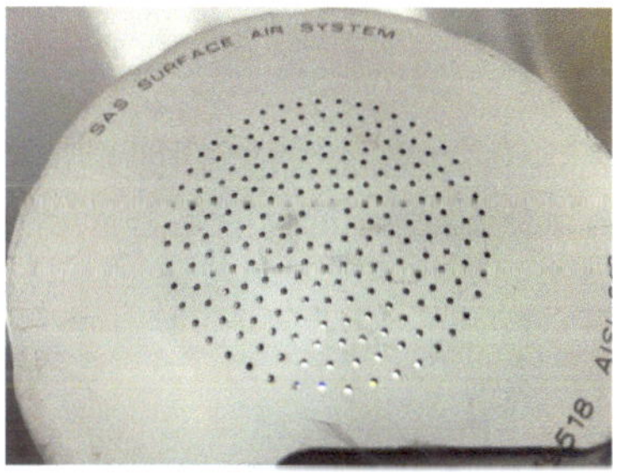

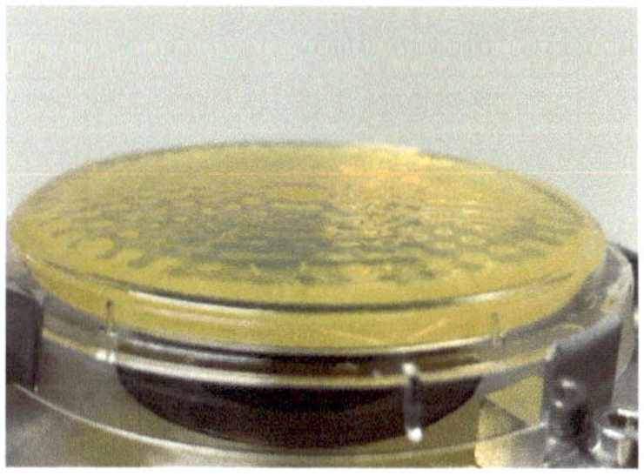

Impaction air samplers have sampling heads that contain holes through which the air is drawn into the air sampler. The air impacts the media surface, depositing any microorganisms that may be present. After sampling the media surface is noticeably dimpled, indicating where the air impacted the media surface.

Photos courtesy of Pure Microbiology, LLC

Surface Sampling

Surface samples are collected with plates, paddles, slides, or swabs. These devices must have a raised, convex surface. Contact plates are the most used device because depending on the air sampler used, the same plate type can be used to collect both viable air and surface samples. Since the media surface will contact a surface in the controlled environment, it is necessary to clean and disinfect the surface after collection to remove any media residue that may be left on the surface. To collect a surface sample using a contact plate:

1. Remove the lid from the plate
2. Collect the sample using a rolling motion
3. Replate the lid onto the plate
4. Clean and disinfect the sampled area

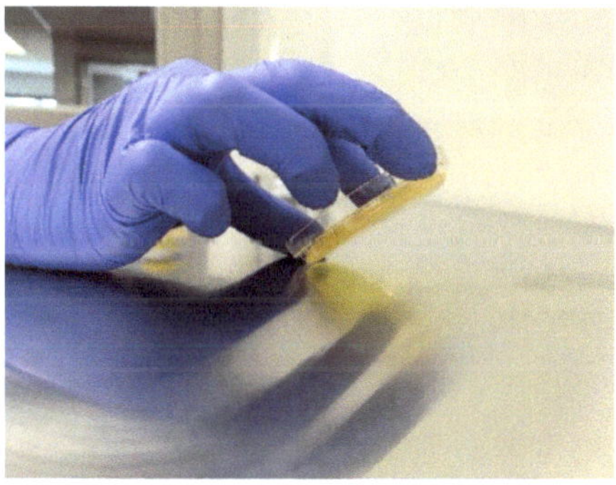

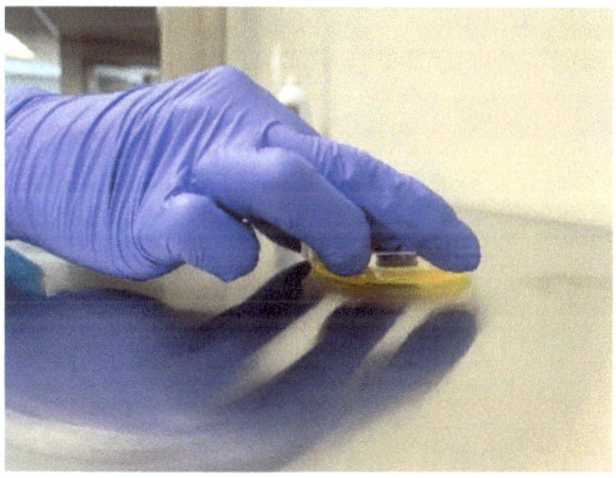

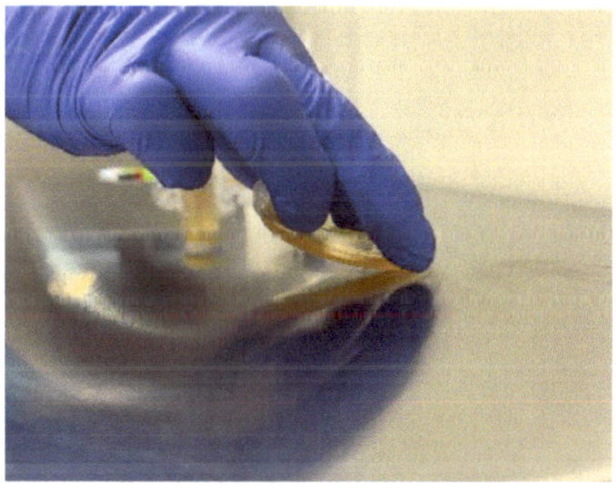

This series depicts the uni-directional rolling motion used to collect surface samples.

Performing a Viable Sampling Session

Each organization will have its own procedures for preparing to sample and completing the sampling session. There are some general principles that all organizations will follow when preparing to sample and completing the sampling session.

Preparing to Sample

1. Plan for dynamic conditions
   a. This is a chapter requirement for air and surface sampling
   b. There must be activity in each PEC
2. Plan for sample shipment, if sending the samples to a contract lab for incubation
   a. Ship the samples overnight for next-day delivery
   b. Sampling may need to be done earlier in the day, depending on the shipping deadline
   c. Confirm the necessary shipping materials are available
3. Plan for sample analysis
   a. If you or your lab does not have weekend hours, the day of sampling needs to be considered to ensure samples do not need to be analyzed during the weekend
4. Obtain the sampling plan
   a. Consider laminating it
   b. It should include sample locations and a list of specific places to sample
5. Prepare media
   a. Verify the media is within the expiration date
   b. If it is refrigerated, allow it to come to room temperature
   c. Ensure there is enough media to sample the required locations and for controls, if necessary
6. Gather all needed supplies
7. Transfer supplies according to facility SOPs

Sample Collection

1. Identify a work area and wipe the surface with sterile 70% IPA
2. For media that will be used in the PEC, it is recommended to open the media in the PEC
   a. It is not recommended to wipe media plates with sterile 70% IPA to transfer them into the PEC. This could cause false negative results if the sterile 70% IPA enters the plate
3. Follow the general sampling order of cleanest to dirtiest
   a. When collecting air samples, wipe the air sampler with sterile 70% IPA before placing into a PEC
4. Be sure to not remove the lid from the plate until collecting the sample
5. Sanitize gloves frequently with sterile 70% IPA
6. When collecting air samples, load the air sampler in the area where the sample will be collected
   a. For example, do not load the air sample in a PEC, and then move the air sampler to the designated sample collection location in the ISO Class 7 space
7. If using locking lid plates, lock the lids after sample collection
8. Label samples on the base of the plate using a marker or label
   a. When labeling by hand, write along the edge of the base of the plate
   b. Label PEC samples outside of the PEC
9. Stay organized by placing collected samples in a bin
10. If a plate is compromised during sampling, mark it as such and discard the plate outside of the clean room suite or SCA
11. Document the necessary information as samples are collected

Sample Session Completion

1. Before exiting the compounding area, confirm all samples were collected along with decontamination materials and equipment if sampling was done in a containment SEC. Do not decontaminate the samples.
2. When using plates without locking lids, use 2 small pieces of tape to secure the lid
3. Incubate samples if incubation is done in-house
4. When shipping samples to a lab:
   a. Complete the chain of custody (COC)
   b. Place the samples in sterile bags
   c. Follow the lab's guidance for shipping
   d. Ship overnight for next-day delivery

Sample Incubation and Analysis

The viable air and surface samples must be incubated for a specified period of time. The incubator's temperature must be monitored throughout the process, either by using a continuous recording device or manual documentation, the results must be reviewed, and the review must be documented.[4] To meet the required incubation parameters of USP <797>, 2 incubators are required and they must be located outside of the sterile compounding area.[4]

Exhibit 5

Recommended Incubation for the Collection of 1 Sample of TSA at Each Sample Location

Stage 1		
30-35 °C	48 hours - 4 days	Read samples

Stage 2		
20-25 °C	5 - 7 days	Read samples

Exhibit 6

Recommended Incubation for the Collection of 1 Sample of TSA and 1 Sample of TSA or Fungal Media at Each Sample Location

TSA		
30-35 °C	48 hours - 4 days	Read samples

Transfer TSA if fungal media was used		
20-20 °C	5 - 7 days	Read samples

TSA or fungal media		
20-25 °C	5 - 7 days	Read samples

Both viable air and surface samples are incubated at 2 temperatures. The incubation procedure depends on whether 1 or 2 samples were collected at each location. The chapter provides incubation parameters and specifies that the samples must be inverted during incubation. If 1 sample is collected at each sample location, it is incubated at 30-35°C for at least 48 hours and then transferred to 20-25°C for at least 5 days. If 2 samples are collected at each location, 1 sample is incubated at 30-35 °C for at least 48 hours and the other sample is incubated at 20-25 °C for at least 5 days.[4] One concern with this procedure is that the incubation time is not capped. Media left in the incubator too long can desiccate and result in the recovered microorganisms no longer being identifiable. Exhibits 5 and 6 describe the recommended incubation and analysis of samples for the single plate and dual plate methods to ensure sample integrity. You will note that the best practice incubation for the dual plate method includes transferring the TSA to 20-25 °C if a fungal medium was used. This allows for a more complete picture of the microorganisms recovered from the sterile compounding area.

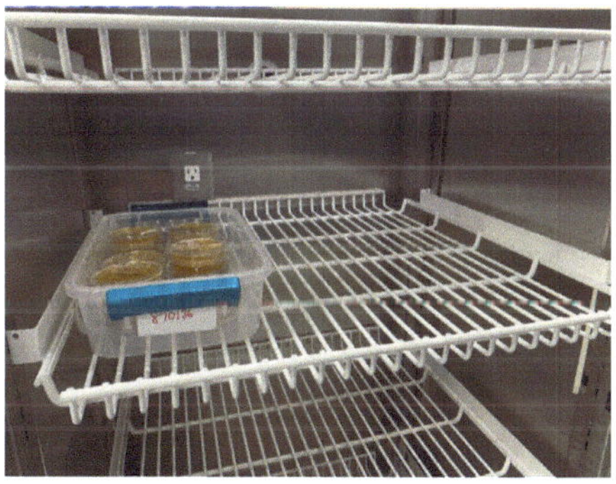

Photo courtesy of Pure Microbiology, LLC

Practical Solution: *Place samples from the same sampling session in a bin for incubation. This keeps the incubator organized and prevents sample mix-ups. It also prevents stacks of samples from being accidentally knocked over during incubation. Bins can be labeled with a*

Why are 2 temperatures needed?

Different microorganisms grow at different temperatures and if we don't provide the temperatures they need, we may miss contamination. Clean room isolates need dual incubation, ideally at 30-35°C and 20-25°C. The reason for this is because the compounding area has 2 climates. The first is the environmental temperature of the compounding area which is 20-25°C. The second is the temperature of human skin, which is approximately 30°C.

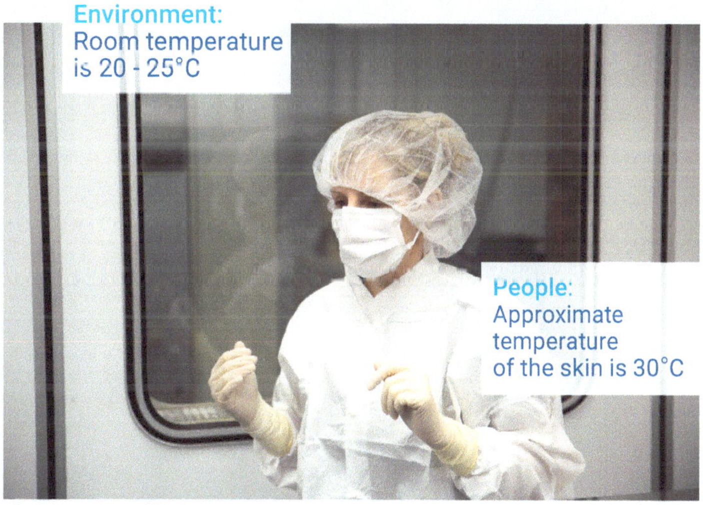

Photo courtesy of Contec, Inc.

handwritten or printed label that includes the date and types of samples (e.g. monthly sampling, investigative sampling, etc.).

After the appropriate incubation, the growth on the samples is counted and the results are compared to the action levels. If 2 samples were collected in each location, the action levels are applied to each sample. The resulting count is not added together. For example, for surface sampling in the ISO Class 7 buffer room, the TSA plate has 6 CFU and the MEA plate has 2 CFU. Since the action level for the area is >5 CFU/plate, the TSA plate is exceeded while the MEA plate is acceptable. But since the TSA sample for the location was exceeded, both samples must be collected after the appropriate corrective actions are implemented.

Sterile compounding personnel can read viable samples, but they must be trained and deemed competent to do so. When counting colonies:

1. Wear gloves and sanitize often with 70% IPA.
2. Look at the colonies before you start counting.
3. Mark the base of the plate with a dot using a permanent marker.
4. If growth is noted IN the agar, contact the manufacturer and start an investigation.
5. If the plate has more than 250 CFU, document the result as Too Numerous to Count (TNTC).
6. Be careful reading air samples, as the dimpling on the agar surface can make small colonies hard to see.
7. Count a spreading colony as 1 CFU.
8. If a colony is growing on top of another, count them as 2 CFU.
9. Include obvious contamination in the count and note on the data sheet.

Practical Solution: *The chapter only requires identification of growth on samples that exceeded the stated action level. Remember that the chapter is a minimum standard and facilities can choose to do more. Consider identifying all growth recovered in the PEC regardless of the number of CFUs recovered. This information can be used to identify risk points in the process and reduce the chances of contamination in the future.*

Investigating Exceeded Action Levels

Exceeded action levels are going to happen and that's okay! They force sterile compounding organizations to look at their processes and implement improvements when necessary. Think of them as part of the quality improvement process.

USP <797> requires an investigation in the event of an exceeded action level, but it does not provide specific guidance on how to investigate. However, some general guidance is offered. The chapter specifies the following[1]:

- The cause of the excursion must be investigated, and corrective action must be taken.
- Data collected in response to corrective actions must be reviewed to confirm that the actions taken have been effective.
- The corrective action plan must be dependent on the colony forming unit (CFU) count and the microorganism recovered.
- The extent of the investigation should be consistent with the deviation and should include an evaluation of trends.
- The corrective action plan must be documented.
- If levels measured during viable air or surface sampling exceed the prescribed levels, an attempt must be made to identify any microorganism recovered to the genus level with the assistance of a microbiologist.

It is necessary to create an SOP that defines how to investigate. The SOP needs to provide an outline of what is to be included in the investigation yet needs to be flexible so that the sterile compounding organization can investigate the excursion appropriately. This is because the "next steps depend on several factors as investigations are unique to every excursion type and every organization."[6] In some investigations, the data will clearly indicate that immediate corrective actions are required. But in other situations, it may be best to monitor the situation, collect more data, and get a better understanding of the situation before taking any action.[6] As an example, 50 CFU/m^3 recovered on an air sample in a PEC will warrant extensive immediate corrective action, while the recovery of 11 CFU/m^3 in an ISO Class 7 anteroom may simply need verification of procedures and to be resampled.

Practical Solution: *Performing an exceeded action level investigation can be stressful and you'll likely feel pressured to resolve the issue as quickly as possible. USP <797> requires that the colonies on the exceeded sample be identified to the genus level; however, identifying the recovered growth to the species level provides greater insight to the possible source, and may bring the investigation to a close more quickly.*

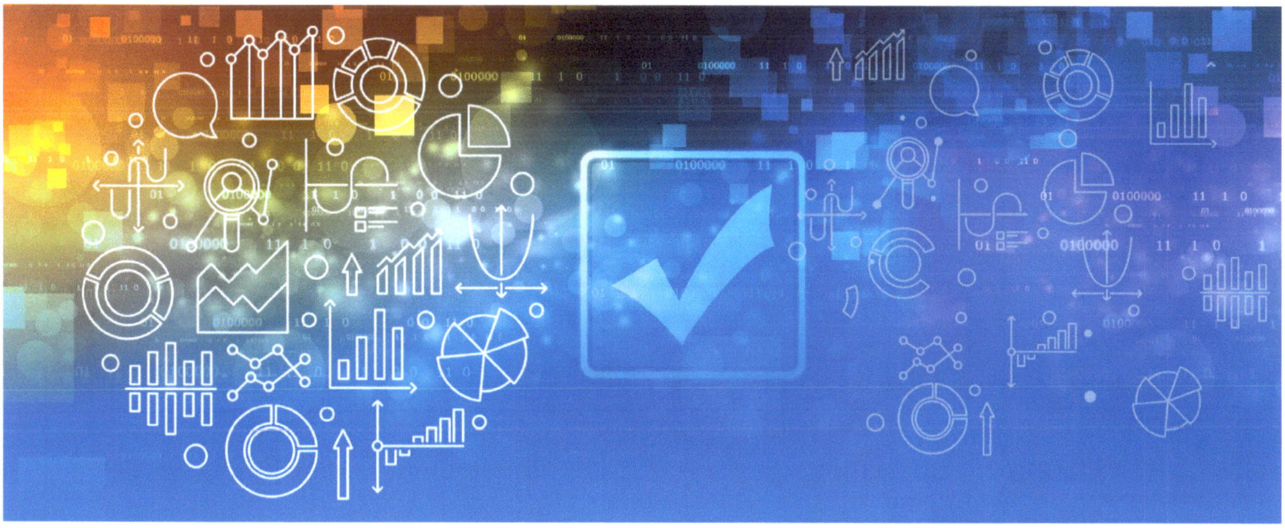

Data Trending

Data trending is a USP <797> chapter requirement. Trending detects adverse trends, determines the typical microbial counts, and creates a proactive approach to contamination control. This ensures an adequate and continued microbial state of control. Trending also identifies:

- If contamination control methods are effective
- Changes in the quantity and types of organisms
- The need to establish and reevaluate action levels

But trending is only effective if there are enough data points. Viable air sampling every 6 months does not produce enough data to effectively ensure the desired state of control. Also be sure that the sampling locations are kept consistent from session to session, as this could also affect the value of the data. When evaluating data, look for:

- Upward or downward trends
- Fluctuations
- Migration of microorganisms to other areas
- Correlation of microorganisms with any failed media fill testing or gloved fingertip sampling
- Association with certain personnel or shifts
- Correlation with changes to facility operations, such as cleaning practices, garbing, and movement of equipment within PEC and clean room suite

Practical Solution: *There are a variety of data trending options. A spreadsheet program is a cost-effective, readily available solution. There are also general trending and viable sampling-specific software programs available. In some cases, sampling vendors or contract testing labs provide data trending. Talk with them to see what they offer.*

Summary

Viable sampling is a valuable tool that provides insight into the sterile compounding area's state of microbial control. Sterile compounding organizations must implement a robust viable sampling program that is appropriately documented. As part of the development, a risk-based approach should be used to select sample locations to ensure the data generated is meaningful. If needed, work with the necessary vendors for sample collection and incubation. The success of the viable sampling program is dependent on staff dedication to data review and the implementation of corrective actions, even if action levels were not exceeded.

References

1. Roth, A. Environmental Monitoring in the Clean Room. INFUSION. Sept/Oct 2017.
2. United States Pharmacopeia. <1116> Microbial Evaluation of Clean rooms and Other Controlled Environments. USP43-NF38.
3. Pure Microbiology. Viable Sampling Challenges and Limitations. July 19, 2022.
4. United States Pharmacopeia. <797> Pharmaceutical Compounding—Sterile Preparations. Revision. November 2022.
5. Controlled Environment Testing Association. CAG-009 Viable Environmental Monitoring for Sterile Compounding Facilities. 2020.
6. Roth, A. Remediating Environmental Monitoring Excursions. *Pharmacy Purchasing & Products.* May 2022 – Vol. 19 No. 5

Summary: Viable Air and Surface Sampling

Viable Sampling Program Checklist

1. Documentation of monitoring procedures, test results, and corrective actions
    a. Diagram of the sampling locations
    b. Procedures for collecting samples
    c. Frequency of sampling
    d. Size of samples
    e. Time of day of sampling in relation to activities in the compounding area
    f. Action levels
2. Maintenance of all associated records
3. Review of data collected in response to corrective actions to verify the actions taken were effective
4. Collection of impaction air samples and surface samples
5. Analysis of data to detect trends

Media Checklist

1. Viable air – TSA in either a settle plate or contact plate based on the air sampler used
2. Surface – TSA with lecithin and polysorbate 80 plates
3. Irradiated
4. Double or tripple bagged
5. Storage conditions appropriate for your facility
6. Reasonable expiration date

Recommended Viable Air and Surface Locations Based on ISO Classification

ISO Class	Viable Air Samples	Surface Samples
5	• 1 sample in the DCA • If the PEC has more than 1 DCA, both must be sampled • DCA of the main chamber of a RABS • Transfer chamber of a RABS (if it is HEPA purged and classified as class 5)	• 1 sample in the DCA* • DCA of the main chamber of a RABS • Transfer chamber of a RABS • Equipment housed in the PEC
7	• Directly outside the PEC where the staff are located • By workstations • Any area that has higher particle counts • By the pass-through chamber door	• Many options, some provide better data on the state of control than others • Staging or work areas near the PEC carts and tables • Interior of the pass-through chamber* • Refrigerators • Shelving • Workflow systems
8	• On the clean side of the line of demarcation • By workstations • Any area that has higher particle counts • By the pass-through chamber door if there is a pass-through chamber to the unclassified space	

* USP <797> required sample location

Viable Air Sample Collection

1. Remove sampling head
2. Load plate
3. Remove lid and place sampling head
4. Start the air sampler
5. When complete, remove the head
6. Check for dimpling, place the plate lid
7. Remove the plate

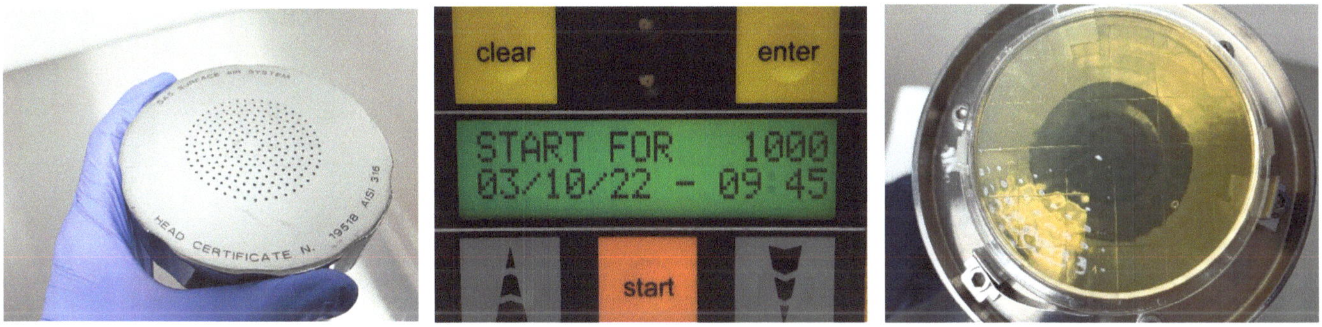

Photos courtesy of Pure Microbiology, LLC

Surface Sample Collection

1. Remove the lid of the plate
2. Place the edge of the plate on the surface to be sampled
3. Collect the sample using a rolling motion
4. Return the lid to the plate
5. Clean and disinfect the sampled area

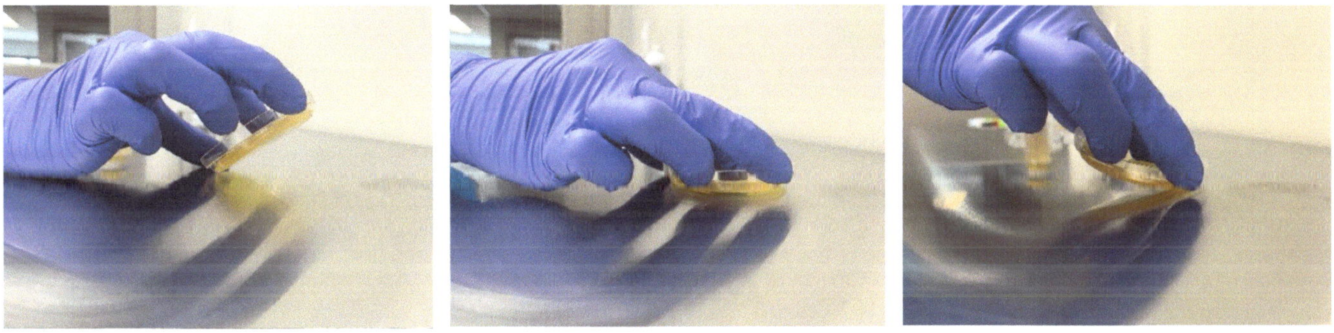

Photos courtesy of Pure Microbiology, LLC

UNIT 7

Preparation, Handling, Storage, Packaging, and Transport of CSPs

The preparation of a CSP is a complex process that blends contamination control, aseptic technique, and quality assurance/control principles. To ensure CSPs are properly prepared, supplies, components, and equipment must meet certain criteria identified in USP General Chapter <797>. The chapter also addresses the use of pharmacy bulk packages, commercially available single- and multiple-dose containers, and compounded single- and multiple-dose containers. Depending on the compounding process, sterilization or depyrogenation may be required, both of which must be tightly controlled to produce repeatable results. In this unit, the general life cycle of a CSP, from preparation through transport, is discussed. Quality-related processes, such as labeling and release testing, are included in Unit 9 Quality Management in Sterile Compounding.

Supplies

The compounding process dictates the supplies needed for safe preparation of CSPs. As a provider of infusion medications, you are likely performing sterile-to-sterile compounding and using all commercially available sterile supplies. These supplies would likely include needles, syringes, and tubing sets. However, some might have a need to provide CSPs that require non sterile to sterile compounding, involving items like beakers and utensils.

In either case, USP <797> indicates that supplies used in compounding *"should be of suitable composition such that the surfaces that contact components are not reactive or sorptive."*[1] Although this is a should statement, ideally each sterile compounding organization carefully evaluates supplies for compatibility with the drug components. The chapter also requires that any supplies in direct contact with the CSP must be sterile and depyrogenated.[1] These processes are discussed in greater detail later in this unit.

Components

USP <797> defines a component as *"any ingredient used in the compounding of a preparation, including any active ingredient, added substance, or conventionally manufactured product."*[1] Each organization must develop SOPs that address a variety of activities related to components and container closures, including:

- Selection
- Receipt
- Evaluation
- Handling
- Storage
- Documentation

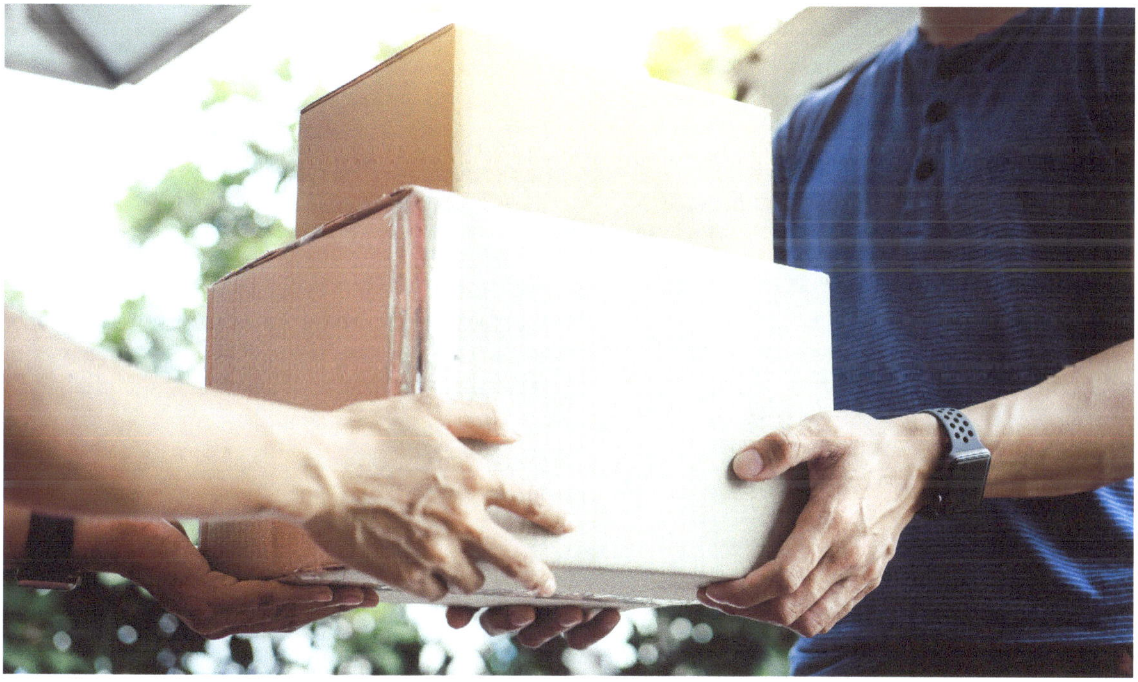

Think about your SOPs. Do they address all these component-related activities? If not, how could the SOPs be improved?

Component Selection

A safe medication starts with the right components. Ideally, a conventionally manufactured sterile product is used, but in some cases, this may not be an option, based on the CSP prepared.[1] This leaves it to the sterile compounding organization to verify that components are appropriate for use. Fortunately, USP <797> provides guidance on the selection of active pharmaceutical ingredient (API) and other components. Exhibit 1 compares USP expectations for API and other components.

Exhibit 1
Comparison of USP Expectations for API and Other Components[1]

API	Other Components
Must comply with the criteria in the *USP–NF* monograph, if one exists	**Must** comply with the criteria in the *USP–NF* monograph, if one exists
Must have a COA indicating the API meets the required specifications	**Must** be accompanied by a COA or labeling that indicates the component meets the required specifications
Must be obtained from an FDA-registered facility	**Should be** obtained from an FDA-registered facility

There may be instances where a component, other than an API, cannot be purchased from an FDA-registered facility. It is then the responsibility of the designated person(s) to select a component from an acceptable and reliable source, verifying the identity, strength, purity, and quality of the ingredients. This verification could be through visual inspection, evaluation of a COA supplied by the manufacturer, or analytical testing of the component to confirm conformance with the COA or other specifications.

Practical Solution: *Vetting a manufacturer or distributor not registered with the FDA – If you are left with no other choice but to purchase components, other than API, from a facility not registered with the FDA, USP provides 2 chapters that review things to look for to be sure you are getting a quality product. USP <1078> Good Manufacturing Practice for Bulk Pharmaceutical Excipients details methods, facilities, and controls used to ensure the excipient meets the expected quality, purity, safety, and suitability. USP <1197> Good Distribution Practices for Bulk Pharmaceutical Excipients provides guidance on the expected quality management systems for those who are manufacturers, distributors, brokers, suppliers, traders, transporters, forwarding agents, and re-packagers of excipients.*

The quality of APIs and other components matters! The chapter **requires** a suitability evaluation of all APIs and other components used in preparation of CSPs. Review labels for statements like "not for pharmaceutical use," "not for injectable use," or "not for human use." If these or an equivalent statement is noted, the API or other component must not be used to compound. Also, be sure you are using at least a USP/NF grade chemical and not something that is graded as "laboratory," "purified," or "technical."[2]

The chapter includes containers and container closure systems under components. A COA must accompany every lot of commercially available sterile, depyrogenated containers and closures, indicating the items meet the expected specifications for sterility and endotoxin. If commercially available sterile, depyrogenated items are not an option, these processes can be performed by the sterile compounding organization, as long as the efficacy of the processes are established and documented. USP <1228> Depyrogenation and USP <1229> Sterilization of Compendial Articles provides more information on establishing the effectiveness of sterilization and depyrogenation processes.

Component Receipt

Receiving components is a key step in CSP quality assurance. Organizational SOPs need to clearly define the process and documentation requirements, so components are evaluated the same way every time, regardless of who receives the items.

When receiving a lot of a component, examine the packaging for any evidence of damage, deterioration, temperature excursions, and other quality issues. If acceptable, verify the labeling and check for an expiration date. For components without a vendor's expiration date, the sterile compounding facility must assign one. The chapter requires that the date does not exceed 1 year after receipt. Write the designated expiration date and the date received on the component.[1]

There will be times when a component is received and is found to be unacceptable for use. These components must be rejected. As part of this process the components are labeled as "rejected" and are quarantined. Depending on the issue with the components, it may be necessary to contact the distributor or manufacturer. Based on the outcome of that correspondence, the components may need to be returned. If not, the components will require proper disposal. As part of quality assurance practices, an investigation into other lots of that component from that vendor is required to confirm other lots do not have the same issue.

Exhibit 2
Steps in Receiving a Component

Examine packaging

↓

Confirm the condition of the component is acceptable

↓

Verify labeling

↓

Check for an expiration date, assign if needed

↓

Mark the component with the received date

↓

Reject, label, and segregate unacceptable components

↓

Examine other lots from that vendor for the same issue

Practical Solution: *The chapter defines requirements for receiving components. Consideration should be given to including all compounding supplies in the receiving process. Receiving personnel should confirm that the item ordered was the item received. The packaging integrity, expiration date, and sterilization status should also be verified.*

Component Handling and Storage

USP <797> requires that components are "handled and stored in a manner that prevents contamination, mix-ups, and deterioration."[1] How do you accomplish this in your organization? Do you have a component handling and storage policy that all staff are trained on?

Contamination risks can be managed by storing components in clean, well-maintained areas. These areas should be routinely cleaned and be part of a pest control program. Components should be stored off the floor and left in plastic overwraps to protect the contents from dust and other contamination risks.

The Institute for Safe Medication Practices (ISMP) provides a variety of strategies to manage medication mix-ups during procurement, prescribing, storage, dispensing and administration. Storage recommendations for medications with problematic, error-prone, look-alike and/or sound-alike names in the pharmacy include:[3]

- Storing these medications in separate physical locations away from each other
- Communicating changes in the location of a problematic product through signage, if automated storage technologies are not used
- Changing the appearance of look-alike medication names on shelves and bins
    - Tall man letters
    - Bold font
    - Different colored font
    - Highlighting or circling critical differentiating information
- Reserving auxiliary warning labels for the most problematic look-alike products

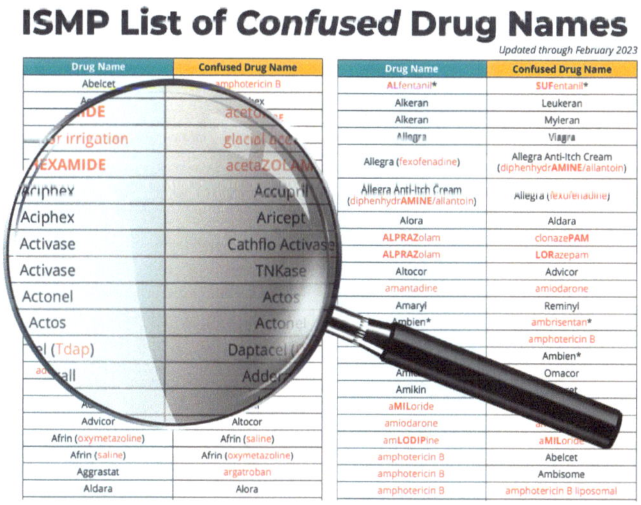

To prevent deterioration of components, they must be stored in closed containers according to the official monograph or supplier/manufacturer instructions. Temperature, humidity, and lighting must all be considered as part of the appropriate storage. As a quality control measure, USP <797> requires that the component storage temperature is monitored to confirm it remains within the acceptable range. This can be accomplished through manual temperature readings daily on days the facility is open, where the result is captured on a log or by a continuous monitoring device, with access to the stored data. It is critical that any monitoring equipment, whether for temperature or humidity, be calibrated or verified for accuracy. Calibrate or verify the monitoring equipment at the frequency recommended by the manufacturer. If a frequency is not provided by the manufacturer, calibrate or verify the monitoring equipment every 12 months.

Component Evaluation

Although a thorough review of components is performed during receipt, it is the responsibility of compounding personnel to evaluate all components before they are used in a sterile preparation. The following must be included in this evaluation:

- Correct identity
- Appropriate quality
- Within expiry date
- Appropriate storage conditions
- Package integrity
- Appearance
- Aroma
- Texture

There are a variety of documents that can help you evaluate components before use. These include:

- Prescription or medication order
- Compounding record
- Master formulation record, if used
- Vendor label(s)
- COA(s) of API(s) and other component(s)
- Product labeling of any conventionally manufactured sterile products
- Labeling of CSP(s)
- Documentation of the compounding facility's storage conditions and practices

How does your organization perform this task and document it?

In addition to evaluating components, sterile containers and closures must be visually inspected. During this inspection, look for defects or other issues that could compromise sterility. Also, confirm the sterile containers and closures are suitable for their intended use. If a component, container, or closures system is found to be unsuitable for use, a similar policy to component receipt must be in place.

Equipment

Different pieces of equipment are essential to sterile compounding. These include primary engineering controls (PECs), automated compounding devices (ACDs), balances, and workflow management systems. There are several things to consider when choosing a piece of equipment. Exhibit 3 lists these considerations.

Exhibit 3
Considerations for Choosing a Piece of Equipment

Composition	Not only does the equipment need to be easily cleanable, but if it contacts components, it should also be of suitable composition as to not be reactive or sorptive.
Function	Equipment must operate properly and within the required performance parameters.
Placement	This could be within the facility or within the PEC. In either case the placement must facilitate workflow and proper compounding technique in your facility.
Calibration / Certification	Equipment must be calibrated as required by the manufacturer and certified every 6 months as defined by USP <797>. Be prepared to maintain these schedules.
Maintenance	Ongoing preventive maintence is essential to the long-term function of the equipment. Perform maintenance tasks as required by the manufacturer.
Cleaning	Although USP <797> provides cleaning requirements, the equipment manufacturer will provide cleaning recommendations, particularly in regards to agents. Be sure the cleaning agent you chose is compatible with the equipment surfaces and electronics.

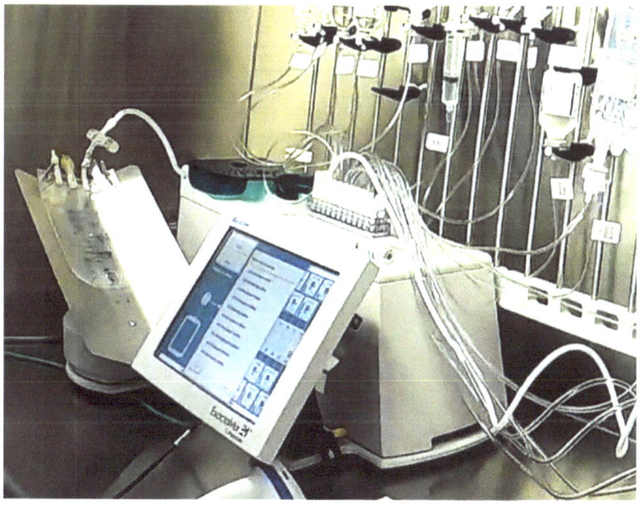

Photo courtesy of Optum

Placement of equipment in the PEC must be carefully considered. Large pieces of equipment, like a TPN compounder, will affect the unidirectional airflow of the PEC and impact first air delivery to critical sites.

Those in the home infusion industry are likely to use ACDs daily. These devices are particularly valuable because they are designed to deliver specific volumes through computerized control. To ensure the continued effectiveness and safety of these devices, USP <797> requires compounding personnel to:[1]

1. Conduct an accuracy assessment before use, every day the equipment is used
2. Maintain a daily record of the accuracy measurements on the days of used
3. Implement corrective actions if accuracy measurements are not as expected

As with any compounding-related activity, a facility must have SOPs in place for the use, calibration, maintenance, and cleaning for every piece of equipment. There must also be a system in place to document these activities.

Preparation

USP <797> does not provide explicit detail on how to prepare a CSP. These processes are developed internally and are documented in facility SOPs and in master formulation records. The chapter instead provides information on the use of conventionally manufactured products and CSPs as components, as well as safety and contamination control considerations.

Certain compounding activities, such as weighing or manipulating, could generate airborne chemical particles. It is the responsibility of the sterile compounding facility to assess these activities, based on its SOPs, and determine if there is a personnel exposure or CSP contamination risk. If so, these activities can be performed in a PEC or other closed-system processing device. The assessment must be documented and retained according to facility procedures.

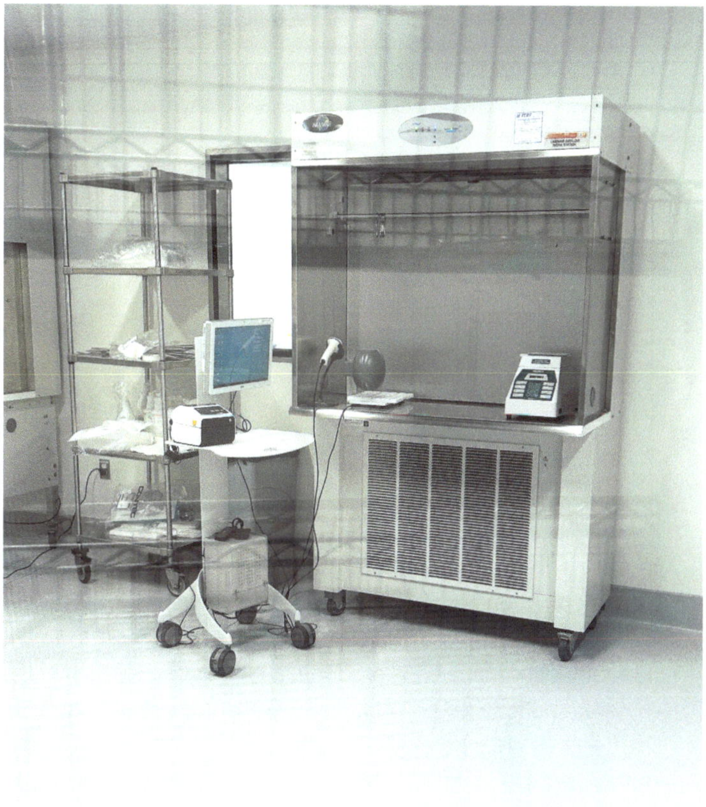

Photo courtesy of Yale New Haven Health System

Conventionally Manufactured Products

The chapter discusses the use of 3 conventionally manufactured products: single-dose containers, multiple-dose containers, and pharmacy bulk packages.

A single-dose container is a container closure system that holds a sterile medication for parenteral administration that is not required to meet the criteria of USP <51> Antimicrobial Effectiveness Testing.[1] Although these containers are designated as "single-dose," they often contain multiple doses of medication. To reduce medication waste, the chapter provides an avenue to retain the container and utilize the additional medication. If a single-dose container is entered or punctured in only ISO Class 5 air, *"it may be used up to 12 hours after the initial entry or puncture as long as the storage requirements during that 12-hour period are maintained."*[1] This means that if the single-dose container requires refrigeration, the container can be removed from the PEC and transferred to a refrigerator for storage until it is needed again, up until 12 hours from initial entry. This does not apply to single-dose ampules, which must not be stored for any period of time.

Exhibit 4

A Comparison of Conventionally Manufactured Products Used in Sterile Compounding[1]

	Single-Dose	Multiple-Dose	Pharmacy Bulk Package
Definition	A container of sterile medication for parenteral administration that is designed for use with a single patient as a single injection/infusion. It usually does not contain a preservative.	A container of sterile medication for parenteral administration that is designed to contain more than 1 dose of the medication. It is usually required to meet the antimicrobial effectiveness testing criteria.	A conventionally manufactured sterile product for parenteral use that contains many single doses intended for use in a pharmacy admixture program. It may either be used to prepare admixtures for infusion or, through a sterile transfer device, for filling sterile containers.
Entry/Puncture Location	In an ISO Class 5 PEC	Not specified in the chapter	In an ISO Class 5 PEC
Timeframe of Use	12 hours	28 days or as specified by the manufacturer	As specified by the manufacturer

A multiple-dose container contains more than 1 dose of a medication and is usually required to meet USP <51> Antimicrobial Effectiveness Testing. Because the containers of these drug products are designed to be entered multiple times, multiple-dose containers are used longer than the single-dose containers once entered or punctured. Upon initial entry or puncture of the multiple-dose container, it must not be used for more than 28 days or as specified by the manufacturer's label.

What is USP <51>? USP General Chapter <51> Antimicrobial Effectiveness Testing describes testing to demonstrate the effectiveness of antimicrobial preservatives added to drug products. To perform this test, a high concentration of a variety of different microorganisms are added to a drug product. Over time, aliquots of the drug product are removed and tested to determine the microbial count. If the preservative system is effective, the number of microorganisms will be logarithmically reduced over the course of 28 days. The test has defined criteria for bacteria, yeast, and mold. This testing is performed by the manufacturer of the drug product. However, when compounding multiple-dose containers, they are required to meet these test requirements, which requires the services of a contract testing lab.

A pharmacy bulk package contains many single doses intended for use in a pharmacy admixture program. The use of these products is limited to the sterile preparation of admixtures for infusion or for the filling of empty sterile containers, using a sterile transfer device. As with the single-dose container, they must be entered or punctured in ISO Class 5 air. However, the use of the pharmacy bulk package must be according to the manufacturer's labeling.

CSPs as Components

In some cases, the organization may compound CSPs to be used as components in other CSPs. These CSPs to be used as components could be multiple-dose CSPs, single-dose CSPs, and compounded stock solutions. It is critical that the organization minimizes the risk of contamination to the CSPs used as components, ensuring proper storage and handling until use. Using CSPs as components requires additional consideration when assigning BUDs to the final CSP. The BUD of the CSP prepared from 1 or more compounded components may not exceed the shortest BUD of any of the individual starting components.

If you compound a multiple-dose CSP to be used as a component, it must meet the criteria of the antimicrobial effectiveness test and be stored under the conditions upon which its BUD is based. After a multiple-dose CSP is initially entered or punctured, it must not be used for longer than the assigned BUD or 28 days, whichever is shorter.

Single-dose CSPs or CSP stock solutions used as components must be entered or punctured in ISO Class 5 air and must be stored under the conditions upon which its BUD is based. The component CSP may be used for up to 12 hours or its assigned BUD, whichever is shorter.

Sterilization and Depyrogenation

Think about your starting supplies and components and the BUDs assigned to preparations. Do you have a need for sterilization and depyrogenation?

Sterilization is "a process that destroys or eliminates all forms of microbial life."[4] Depyrogenation is "the direct and validated destruction or removal of pyrogens."[5] The definitions for sterilization and depyrogenation appear to be similar, but they are 2 different things. Endotoxin, the pyrogens we are concerned with in the compounding of sterile preparations, are not living. They are a lipopolysaccharide component of the cell wall of gram-negative bacteria.[6] Endotoxin must be destroyed through high heat. These parameters are not typically compatible with a wide variety of CSPs. Therefore, a typical terminal steam sterilization cycle will not destroy endotoxin. Additionally, sterilization by filtration using a 0.2-micron filter will not eliminate endotoxin, as it is usually <0.025 microns in size.[7]

These points emphasize why it's crucial to minimize the introduction of gram-negative bacteria and endotoxin into a presterilized preparation. This is also why the chapter requires injectable compounded preparations prepared using non-sterile components or supplies to be sterilized within 6 hours after completing the preparation to minimize the generation of endotoxins in the CSPs.

USP <797> requires that facilities have terminal sterilization and depyrogenation SOPs in place if these activities are part of your compounding process. These SOPs must include:

- A description of the process
- Temperature parameters
- Pressure parameters, if applicable
- Cycle duration
- Permissible load configurations
- Use of biological indicators, physicochemical indicators, and endotoxin challenge vials (ECVs)

Staff must be trained and competent on all sterilization methods and equipment used by the facility. There must also be a schedule and method for establishing and verifying the effectiveness of the selected terminal sterilization and depyrogenation. This would include the use of indicators and as a best practice at least initial and annual validation of the process. SOPs must also document the cleaning and maintenance of the equipment.

Exhibit 5

Compounding Stock Solutions

1. Reconstitute single-dose vials of commercially available product.

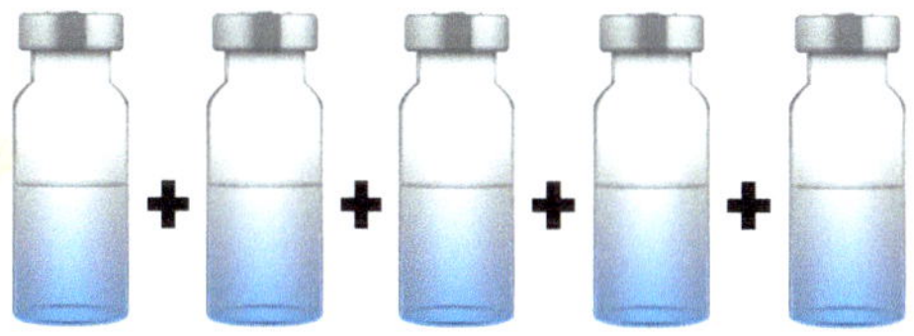

2. Combine single-dose vials into a compounded stock solution.

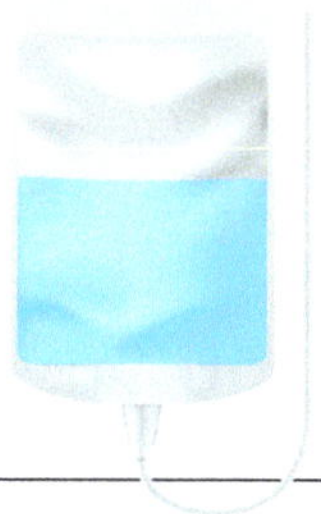

3. Store compounded stock solution according to USP <797> beyond use date (BUD) guidelines.

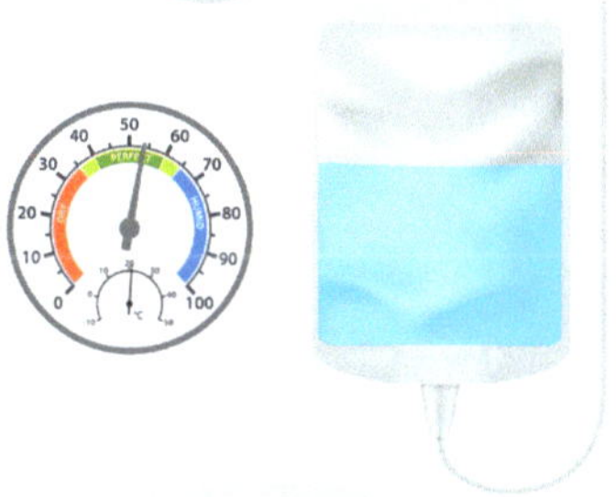

4. Remove stock solution from storage to prepare final compounded sterile preparations (CSPs) in single-dose containers for infusion.

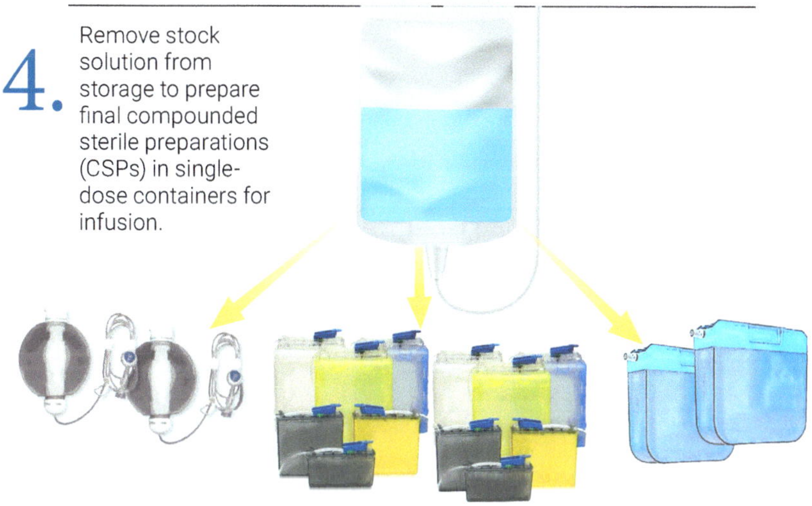

Once stock solution has been used for CSP prep, it must be assigned a 12-hour BUD and labeled appropriately.

5. Assign each of the final CSPs a BUD—based on the shorter BUD of their starting components.

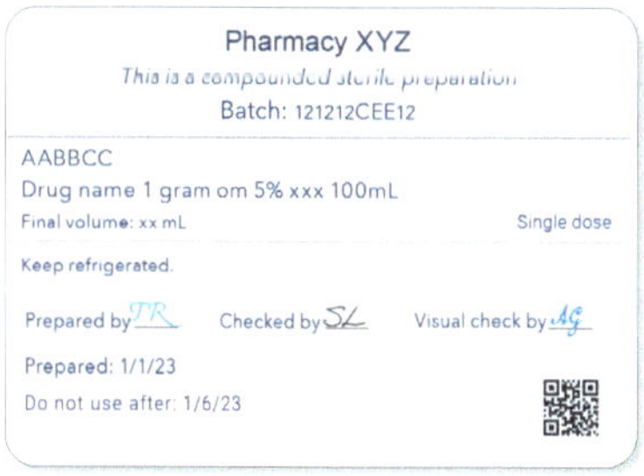

Example: *A compounded stock solution is given a 10-day BUD under refrigeration. It is removed from use after 5 days and used to prepare CSPs. The CSPs can have a BUD of no longer than 5 days, as this was the BUD time remaining on the compounded stock solution.*

***Practical Solution:** Equipment Validation – Sterilization and depyrogenation of equipment are an essential part of the compounding process if starting with non-sterile supplies or components. Validation is the only way to ensure a piece of equipment is working as expected. Even though validation is not explicitly required by the chapter, consider working with a vendor that specializes in equipment validation to be sure your equipment performs accurately and consistently.*

Sterilization

Compounding with non-sterile supplies or components requires some form of sterilization, whether terminal sterilization using a piece of equipment like an autoclave or sterilization by filtration. Terminal sterilization may also be part of your compounding process if BUDs are assigned to CSPs that require it.

Choosing a sterilization method requires research. It is critical that the sterilization method chosen does not degrade the CSP or compromise the packaging integrity.

Sterilization and Depyrogenation USP Chapter Reference List

USP provides numerous guidance chapters on depyrogenation and sterilization. The chapters applicable to a sterile compounding organization, based on compounding methods and BUDs, are listed.

<1228>	Depyrogenation
<1228.1>	Dry Heat Depyrogenation
<1228.3>	Depyrogenation by Filtration
<1228.4>	Depyrogenation by Rinsing
<1228.5>	Endotoxin Indicators for Depyrogenation
<1229>	Sterilization of Compendial Articles
<1229.1>	Steam Sterilization by Direct Contact
<1229.2>	Moist Steam Sterilization of Aqueous Liquids
<1229.4>	Sterilizing Filtration of Liquids
<1229.5>	Biological Indicators for Sterilization
<1229.8>	Dry Heat Sterilization
<1229.9>	Physicochemical Integrators and Indicators for Sterilization

The following must be considered:

- The nature of the component(s)
- Their physical and chemical properties
- The intended container closure system

Terminal sterilization, which includes steam and dry heat, is the preferred sterilization method, if the CSP and container closure system can handle the conditions. Filtration is another option, so long as the suspended drug particles are not removed by the filter.

The reason terminal sterilization is preferred over sterilization by filtration is because the terminal sterilization process is intended to achieve a probability of a non-sterile unit (PNSU) of 10^{-6}. This means that there is a probability of having 1 CSP out of 1 million CSP being non-sterile. Aseptically preparing a CSP, even if using a sterilizing filter, results in a PNSU of 10^{-3} or 1 CSP out of 1000 CSPs being non-sterile.[8]

Probability of a Non-sterile Unit (PNSU)
The probability of an item being non-sterile after it has been exposed to a verified sterilization process.[1]

Excessive particulate matter in CSPs is a concern. The chapter requires that all CSPs sterilized using steam or dry heat have a prefiltration step to remove excessive particulate matter, while CSPs sterilized by filtration only need a prefiltration step when the CSP is known to have excessive particulate matter. Prefiltration is performed using a filter with a pore size of not larger than 1.2 μm.

Sterilization by Steam Heat

Sterilization by steam heat is the process of using saturated steam under pressure to sterilize items, better known as autoclaving. This is the preferred method for terminal sterilization of aqueous CSPs in their final, sealed container closure system. However, if steam sterilization would degrade the CSPs, then an alternate sterilization method needs to be used.

A successful steam sterilization cycle requires all materials to be directly exposed to steam, under adequate pressure, time, and temperature to achieve the expected destruction of microorganisms. The steam is generated using water defined by the manufacturers, which must result in contaminate-free steam. The autoclave must reach the sterilizing temperature and remain at that temperature for the duration of the defined cycle.

The effectiveness of every steam sterilization cycle must be verified and documented with each sterilization run. This verification is performed by including biological indicators with *Geobacillus stearothermophilus* spores and other confirmation methods such as physicochemical indicators or integrators with items being sterilized. Additionally, the cycle temperature and pressure data must be recorded using a calibrated data recorder or chart, so it can be evaluated for deviations from the designated parameters. The date, run, and load configuration used to sterilize a CSP must be documented in the compounding record.

Sterilization by Dry Heat

USP notes that *"Dry heat sterilization is a process utilized for heat-stable items that are unsuited for steam sterilization because of either an absence of water or requirements for absolute dryness following processing."*[11] This sterilization method is usually performed in a calibrated oven, where heated air is evenly distributed throughout the chamber. To achieve a successful dry heat cycle, higher temperatures and longer exposure times than sterilization by steam are required.

A dry heat sterilization cycle is successful when the items in the oven are exposed to the defined temperature for the required length of time. Dry heat sterilization is typically performed in a range of 160-190°C.[11] If lower temperatures are used, USP <797> requires verification of these temperatures according to USP <1229.8> Validation of Dry Heat Sterilization, Biological Indicators. However, full validation of the cycle is ideal, proving both biological and temperature evidence of an appropriate cycle.

Exhibit 6

Comparison of Steam and Dry Heat Sterilization

Steam	Dry Heat
Preferred method if the CSP allows	For items that cannot be sterilized by steam
Saturated steam under pressure	High heat
Exposure time defined through validation, shorter and cooler than dry heat	Exposure time defined through validation, longer and hotter than steam
BI – *Geobacillus stearothermophilus*	BI – *Bacillus atropheus*
Another cycle confirmation method	Another cycle confirmation method

The effectiveness of the dry heat sterilization cycle is verified and documented with each sterilization run using biological indicators of *Bacillus atrophaeus* spores

What are physicochemical indicators and integrators?

Physicochemical indicators and integrators are also known as chemical indicators. ISO 15882 Sterilization of health care products—Chemical indicators—Guidance for Selection, Use, and Interpretation of Results defines chemical indicator as a *"test system that reveals change in one or more pre-defined process variables based on a chemical or physical change resulting from exposure to a process."*[9] In the case of sterilization, these devices are used to monitor whether 1 or more of the defined cycle parameters were met.

Physicochemical indicators provide "an immediate visual confirmation that an item has been exposed to a sterilization process," but it doesn't necessarily mean the temperature or time parameters of the process were met.[10] For example, steam could be generated during an autoclave cycle, but the cycle didn't reach the required temperature. The indicator would still provide visual evidence that steam was produced.

Physicochemical integrators respond "to one or more sterilization process critical parameters, which results in a measurable value that can be correlated to microbial lethality."[10] With these devices there are chemical reactions that occur when all critical cycle parameters are met, resulting in a visual indication of success or failure.

These indicators are an option when confirming the effectiveness of a steam autoclave cycle. Using an integrator as opposed to an indicator will provide assurance that the cycle parameters were met. However, they cannot be used in isolation. Data from the steam autoclave cycle obtained from calibrated instruments must be used in conjunction with indicators and integrators.[10]

and temperature-sensing devices that are connected to calibrated data recorders or charts. The cycle data must be evaluated for deviations. Document the date, run, and load configuration used to sterilize a CSP in the compounding record.

Practical Solution: *Validate Steam and Dry Heat Sterilization Cycles – USP <797> does not require the validation of steam and dry heat sterilization cycles, only the use of biological indicators and other cycle-success confirmation methods. But the chapter does require SOPs to include permissible load configurations and the times and temperatures of the cycles. A load configuration defines how items are placed in the sterilization equipment, how many can be placed, and the liquid volume the items can hold. The only way to know if a load configuration will work consistently is through validation. And you are likely to find that an autoclave load of 20 containers with 500 mL will require a longer cycle time than 50 containers of 100 mL. It is best to validate this up front than through trial and error on CSP loads.*

Sterilization by Filtration

USP <797> defines sterilization by filtration as the *"passage of a gas or liquid through a sterilizing-grade membrane to yield filtrates that are sterile."*[1] Sterilizing filters must be:[1]

- Sterile
- Depyrogenated
- Have a nominal pore size of 0.22 µm or smaller
- Labeled for pharmaceutical use
- Certified by the manufacturer to meet ASTM F838-20 Standard Test Method for Determining Bacterial Retention of Membrane Filters Utilized for Liquid Filtration

It is the responsibility of the designated person to ensure that the filters:[1]

- Are chemically and physically compatible with all ingredients in the CSP
- Are chemically stable at the pressure and temperature conditions that will be used
- Have enough capacity to filter the required volumes
- Used to sterilize CSPs are tested for integrity (bubble point test)

In the event of a failed filter integrity test, an investigation must be conducted. After investigating the cause of the failure, the CSPs prepared with the failed filter must be discarded or refiltered for sterilization not more than 1 additional time using an appropriate filter.

Depyrogenation

Sterile compounding organizations that use glassware, metal, and other thermostable containers in their non-sterile-to-sterile compounding processes must depyrogenate the items using a dry heat depyrogenation oven. The time and temperature necessary for a successful depyrogenation cycle must be established. All possible load configurations must be identified. Initial and annual verification of the cycle is performed using endotoxin challenge vials. Success is defined by achieving ≥3-log reduction in endotoxins. Any changes to the time, temperature, or load configuration of the established cycles, must be verified to confirm effectiveness. All verification activities must be documented. When using the depyrogenation oven, it is necessary to verify that the oven reached the expected temperature and that it stayed at that temperature through the entire depyrogenation cycle. As discussed with other equipment, validation of the depyrogenation process is recommended.

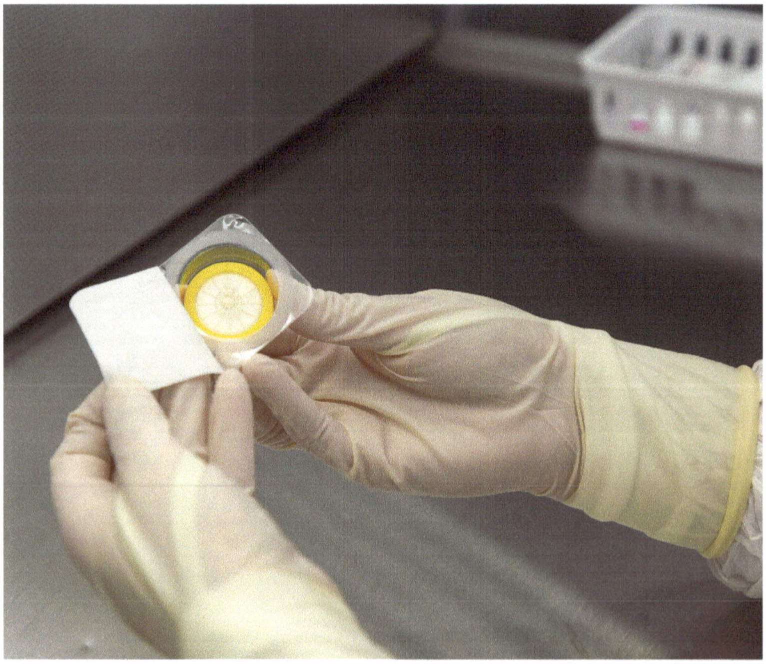

Sterilizing filter

Photo courtesy of Contec, Inc.

Any items used in the compounding process that will contact components or the CSP that are not thermostable must be depyrogenated by rinsing. The rinsing process requires the

> **Can we depyrogenate all items by rinsing? The answer is no.** The chapter specifically indicates that thermostable containers must be subjected to dry heat depyrogenation.[1] There is good reason for this. Depyrogenation by rinsing validation studies have shown that the level of reduction is usually not more than 1-2 logs.[12] Meaning if an item has 1 million endotoxin units on its surface, rinsing may only drop that number to 100,000 or at best 10,000. That's a lot of endotoxin left on the surface that could contaminate a CSP.

use of sterile, non-pyrogenic water such as sterile water for injection or sterile water for irrigation. The items are thoroughly drained or dried immediately before use in compounding.

Handling, Storage, Packaging, and Transporting

Your sterile compounding organization may compound a variety of different CSPs, each requiring different handling, storage, packaging, and transporting requirements. Because of this variety, it is essential to develop SOPs for handling, storing, packaging, and transporting CSPs. Personnel who participate in any of these compounding-related activities must receive documented training.

Handling and Storage

Proper handling and storage ensure the maintenance of CSP quality and package integrity. As part of this maintenance, temperature monitoring of the storage area is performed to confirm CSPs remain in the appropriate temperature range. With the BUDs provided in the chapter, storage conditions can include controlled room temperature storage (20-25°C), refrigerator storage (2-8°C), and freezer storage (-25 – -10 °C).

Choosing the appropriate storage conditions of a CSP is critical to both the stability and microbial sterility of the CSP. Storing CSPs refrigerated or frozen comes with the benefit of slower microbial growth, in the event the CSP was contaminated, but this might not always be an option. The chemical and physical stability of the CSP may be negatively affected at colder conditions. For example, the formulation may precipitate. Another challenge may be the container integrity, especially under frozen conditions. The container closure system must remain intact.

Removing a CSP from cold storage requires consideration. Refrigerated CSPs must be allowed to warm and frozen CSPs must be allowed to thaw in a manner to retain physical and chemical stability, as well as container closure integrity. This process must be designated and documented for each CSP formulation.

It is possible for CSPs to be stored under different conditions before use (frozen, to refrigerated, to room temperature). If this occurs, the storage time of the CSP must not exceed the original BUD based on its labeled storage condition and the BUDs are not additive. Let's look at an example. An aseptically processed CSP prepared from sterile starting component(s) is stored in the freezer, giving it a BUD of 45 days. After 40 days it is removed and thawed in the refrigerator. Once it enters the refrigerator, it now has a maximum BUD of 5 days, instead of the full 10-day refrigerated BUD indicated in Table 11 of USP <797> because it cannot exceed the original BUD of 45 days. Remember, the BUD is not additive. It cannot be stored for 45 days in a freezer, then placed for 10 days in a refrigerator, and then be stored for 4 days at controlled room temperature for a total of 59 days. This would exceed the original 45-day BUD. Also, once a CSP has been stored under a condition that requires a shorter BUD, it must be used within the new timeframe.

Monitoring the temperature of the storage areas is the only way to ensure the necessary storage temperatures are met. The chapter requirements for temperature monitoring include:

- Daily monitoring, either manually or by a continuous recording device
- Documentation of the temperature readings in a temperature log or stored in the continuous temperature recording device
- Retrievable data
- Accuracy verification of the temperature monitoring devices at least every 12 months or as required by the manufacturer
- Detection of temperature excursions

The goal of the sterile compounding facility is to minimize temperature excursions. However, when it is identified that a CSP is exposed to temperatures out of the allowable range, it is the responsibility of a designated person(s) to determine whether the CSP is still safe, efficacious, and appropriate for use. This investigation can be accomplished through literature review or through analytical testing. If there is any evidence suggesting the CSP quality or integrity has been compromised, it must be discarded.

Packaging, Shipping, and Transport

What happens to the CSPs you prepare? Are they given to patients in your facility or sent to other locations? How do you ensure CSPs arrive in an acceptable condition for use?

CSPs may be transported within your facility, to other facilities, or directly to patients. The packaging materials chosen to transport CSPs should protect them from damage, leakage, contamination, degradation, and adsorption, in addition to preventing inadvertent exposure to transport personnel. However, the facility "must select modes of transport that are expected to deliver properly packed CSPs in an undamaged, sterile, and stable condition."[1] The materials selected for shipping and packaging must be based on:

- The CSP specifications
  - Light sensitivity
  - Temperature needs
  - Tamper-evident closures
- Information from vendors
- The mode of transport

As part of the packaging, CSPs that require special handling must include specific handling instructions on the outside of the container.

Packaging Considerations – You likely noticed that the word "should" was used in the discussion regarding packaging materials chosen for transporting CSPs. This is chapter language and although this is not written as a must, the necessary packaging to safely transport CSPs needs to be carefully evaluated. Incidents of CSP issues due to packaging and transport should be reported through some type of feedback mechanism to the designated person, investigated, and corrective action taken.

***Practical Solution:** Shipping Temperature Verification*

Maintaining the temperature of a CSP through the shipping process can be challenging, especially when shipping to areas with temperature extremes. Sterile compounding organizations that ship CSPs should strongly consider performing a study to verify that the packaging chosen can maintain the expected USP storage conditions through the potential shipping options (by pharmacy personnel in a vehicle, through a third-party carrier, by company courier).

1. *Choose the shipping container, cooling method (if required), and packaging material to secure the CSPs in the shipping container.*
2. *Identify worst-case shipping conditions, including the longest period a CSP could be exposed to a temperature extreme.*
3. *Include temperature monitoring devices that measure parameters in accordance with desired temperature ranges tested.*
4. *Test each possible shipping scenario at least 3 times.*
5. *Modify packaging if temperatures are not maintained and retest.*
6. *Maintain the results of these verification procedures.*
7. *Perform additional testing if packaging materials, types of CSPs, storage requirements, or delivery conditions change.*

Summary

Preparation through transport of a CSP requires meticulous planning and evaluation. Choosing the wrong container closure or not properly calibrating a piece of equipment can put a patient at risk. All sterile compounding personnel need a strong foundation in the use of components and supplies, the calibration, use, and maintenance of equipment, and the storage and handling of final CSPs.

References

1. United States Pharmacopeia. <797> Pharmaceutical Compounding—Sterile Preparations. Revision. November 2022.
2. Schieving, A. The Seven Most Common Grades for Chemical and Reagents. *Lab Manager.* November 17, 2017.
3. Institute for Safe Medication Practices. Adopt Strategies to Manage Look-Alike and/or Sound-Alike Medication Name Mix-Ups. Featured Articles. June 2, 2022.
4. Centers for Disease Control and Prevention. Introduction, Methods, Definition of Terms. Guideline for Disinfection and Sterilization in Healthcare Facilities. 2008.
5. United States Pharmacopeia. <1228> Depyrogenation. Official May 18, 2021.
6. Tille PM. Bailey and Scott's Diagnostic Microbiology 14th ed. Page 1079. 2014.
7. United States Pharmacopeia. <1228.3> Depyrogenation by Filtration. Official Dec 1, 2016.
8. von Woedtke T, Kramer A. The limits of sterility assurance. *GMS Krankenhhyg Interdiszip.* 2008;3(3): Doc19. Published 2008 Sep 3.
9. International Organization for Standardization. ISO 15882:2008 Sterilization of health care products – Chemical indicators – Guidance for selection, use and interpretation of results.
10. United States Pharmacopeia. <1229.9> Physicochemical Integrators and Indicators for Sterilization. Official Aug 1, 2016.
11. United States Pharmacopeia. <1229.8> Dry Heat Sterilization. Official May 1, 2018.
12. Agalloco, James P. Depyrogenation by Dilution. PharmTech.com February 20, 2008.

Summary: CSP Preparation, Handling, Storage, Packaging, and Transport

Components are the key to a safe CSP. Use this checklist to ensure your SOPs have everything they need to address component-related activities.

Component-Related SOP Checklist

Selection

- **API**
  - Must comply with the criteria in the *USP–NF* monograph, if one exists
  - Must have a COA indicating the API meets the required specifications
  - Must be obtained from an FDA-registered facility
- **Other components**
  - Must comply with the criteria in the *USP–NF* monograph, if one exists
  - Must be accompanied by a COA or labeling that indicates the component meets the required specifications
  - Should be obtained from an FDA-registered facility
- **Container closure system**
  - COA must accompany every lot of commercially available sterile, depyrogenated containers and closures
  - Sterilization and depyrogenation of container closures performed by the sterile compounding facility must have demonstrated efficacy

Receipt

- Examine packaging
- Confirm the condition of the component is acceptable
- Verify labeling
- Check for an expiration date, assign if needed
- Mark the component with the received date
- Reject, label, and segregate unacceptable components

Handling and Storage

- Must be handled and stored in a manner that prevents contamination, mix-ups, and deterioration
- Stored in closed containers according to the official monograph or supplier/manufacturer instructions
- Temperature, humidity, and lighting must all be considered as part of the appropriate storage

Evaluation

- Before use evaluate the component for:
  - Correct identity
  - Appropriate quality
  - Within expiry date
  - Appropriate storage conditions
  - Package integrity
  - Appearance
  - Aroma
  - Texture

Documentation

- Receipt documentation
- Component marked as received
- COA review
- Evaluation documentation
- Temperature monitoring of component storage

Compounded stock solutions may be a vital part of your compounding process. This infographic depicts how compounded stock solutions are used as CSPs, as defined by USP <797>.

Compounding Stock Solutions

1. Reconstitute single-dose vials of commercially available product.

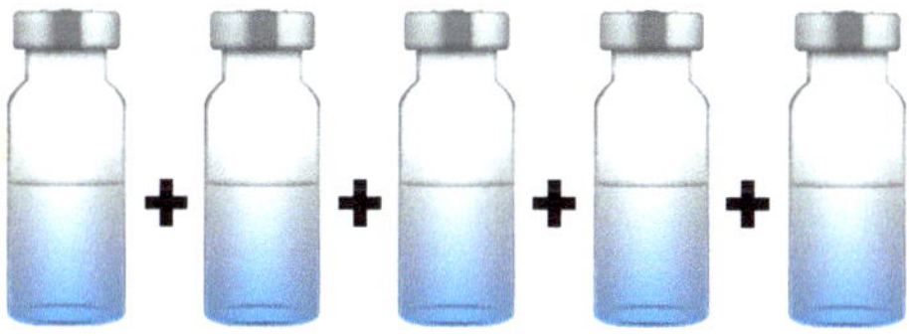

2. Combine single-dose vials into a compounded stock solution.

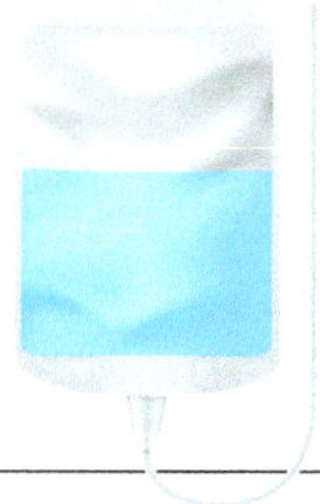

3. Store compounded stock solution according to USP <797> beyond use date (BUD) guidelines.

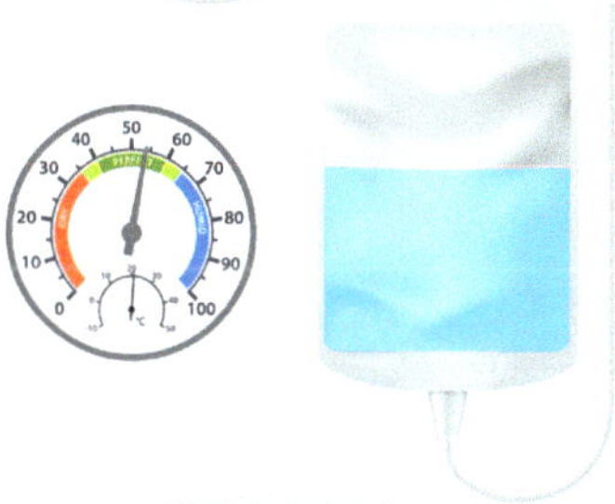

4. Remove stock solution from storage to prepare final compounded sterile preparations (CSPs) in single-dose containers for infusion.

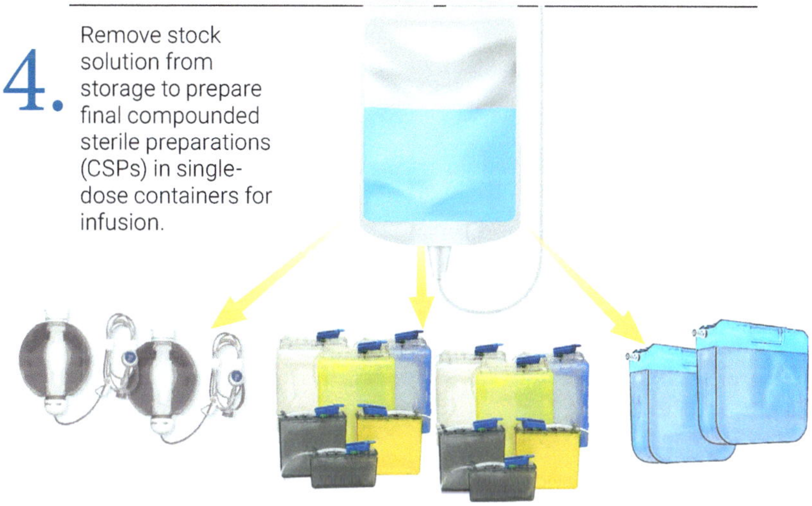

Once stock solution has been used for CSP prep, it must be assigned a 12-hour BUD and labeled appropriately.

5. Assign each of the final CSPs a BUD—based on the shorter BUD of their starting components.

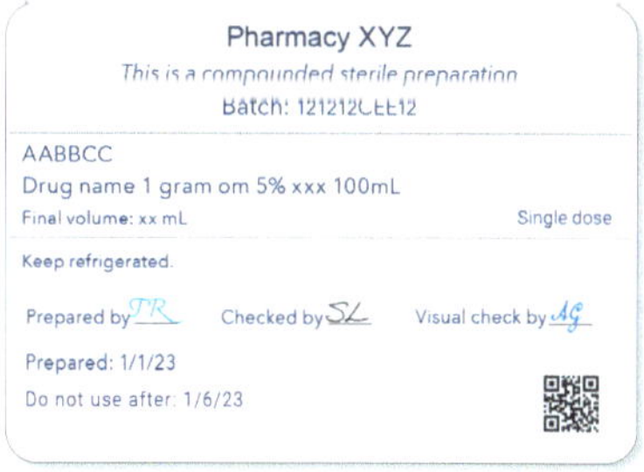

Example: *A compounded stock solution is given a 10-day BUD under refrigeration. It is removed from use after 5 days and used to prepare CSPs. The CSPs can have a BUD of no longer than 5 days, as this was the BUD time remaining on the compounded stock solution.*

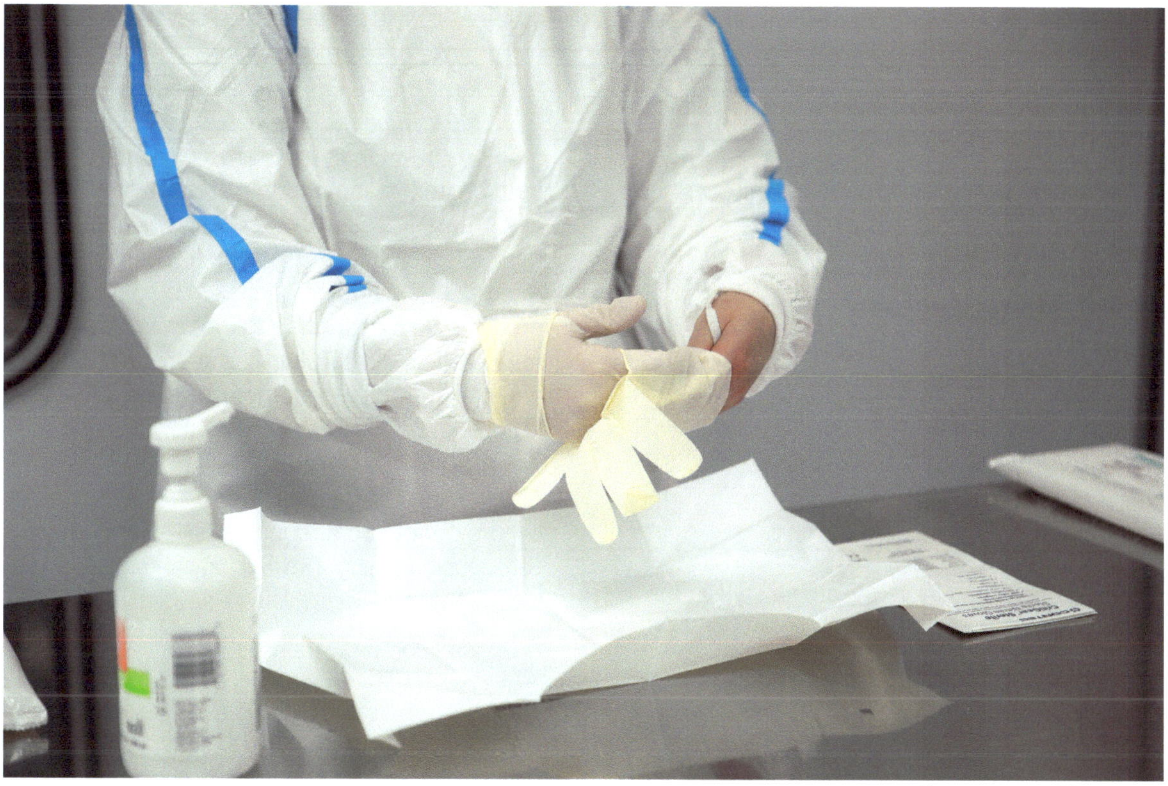

Photo courtesy of Contec, Inc.

UNIT 8

Training and Evaluation

Training and evaluation of sterile compounding personnel is essential to the success of the organization. It takes significant effort to design and implement a robust and effective training program, utilizing the knowledge and experience of numerous staff members, and maybe even external experts. USP General Chapter <797> provides requirements for the minimum training and competency expectations. Ultimately, however, it is the responsibility of the sterile compounding organization to identify the specific training needs based on its operation. This unit reviews the chapter expectations for training and competency assessments and provides practical solutions for the implementation of these expectations.

USP <797> General Training Requirements

Before applying the specific training- and competency-related chapter requirements to a specific organization, it's necessary to have a basic understanding of 6 general requirements.[1]

1. All personnel involved in or having direct oversight of the compounding of CSPs must be initially trained and qualified by demonstrating knowledge and competency in compounding CSPs before being allowed to perform their job functions independently.

2. A designated person(s) ***must*** oversee the training of personnel. This does not mean they are required to perform the training.

3. Personnel involved in or having direct oversight of compounding CSPs ***must*** complete training and competencies initially and at least every 12 months in appropriate sterile compounding principles and practices. Chapter-required competencies are required more frequently.

4. Each compounding facility ***must*** develop a written training program that describes the required training, the frequency of training, and the process for evaluating the performance of individuals involved in preparing CSPs.

5. Training and evaluation of personnel ***must*** be documented.

6. The training program must equip personnel with the appropriate knowledge and train them in the required skills necessary to perform their assigned tasks, and SOPs should specify the training required for such tasks.

To summarize these 6 requirements, the sterile compounding organization must have a written and documented training program, overseen by the designated person, that provides training and qualification of staff in all compounding-related activities they perform. Think about your training and competency program. Does it meet all these general requirements?

Training Program Development

Developing a robust, effective training program can be challenging. Although each organization will have different program needs, in a simplistic view, all training programs should:

1. Provide "the why behind the what"
2. Be based on organizational SOPs
3. Recognize and accept different learning styles and needs
4. Define training components
5. Identify assigned trainers

Let's explore each of these and how they can be incorporated into a training program.

"The Why Behind the What"

USP <797> defines everything a sterile compounding organization must do, with the goal being the safety of the patient. But have you ever read the chapter and asked why a particular requirement exists, wanting an explanation? The same type of question may be asked of your organization's SOPs. Why do we have to perform a task this way? What's the rationale? These types of questions are why it's important to include "the why behind the what" in a training program. Staff who embrace the rationale behind an SOP, help to ensure the preparation of safe medications.[2] They will be doing more than going through the motions.

Training Based on Organizational SOPs

An organization's training program is only as good as its SOPs. Clear, detailed SOPs are the foundation of the training program, ensuring that all work performed in the organization is consistent and capable of providing repeatable results.[2] As SOPs are updated, the training program must also be updated.

Recognition and Acceptance of Different Learning Styles and Needs

When developing the training program, the organization must respect that training takes time. Proper onboarding of new staff members is non-negotiable for the organization's success. Every person has a different learning style and a robust training program will provide different approaches to training as needed to accommodate different learning styles. Those new to sterile compounding will require a longer initial training period than experienced compounders, but both share the same training requirements. There will also be instances where trainees may be struggling with a particular task, such as donning sterile gloves. Alternate training approaches should be provided, like practicing gloving with a trainer outside of the clean room. A less stressful environment might be needed until the individual becomes competent in a skill.

Training Components

The training program must define initial training, which occurs prior to compounding CSPs for human use, and subsequent training. The training program should generally include the following, which are specific to the organization:

- General company training
  - SOPs
  - Mission and goals
  - Human resources expectations
- Pharmacy-specific training
  - SOPs
  - Calculations
  - Equipment and software
- Sterile compounding training
  - SOPs and industry documents
  - Didactic learning
  - Shadowing
  - Practice sessions
  - Personnel testing
  - Annual training and competencies (Be sure to include things like new therapies and SOPS changes to staff's ongoing training.)

USP <797> defines specific training areas that must minimally be completed initially and at least every 12 months. These areas include:[1]

- Hand hygiene and garbing
- Cleaning and disinfection
- Calculations, measuring, and mixing
- Aseptic technique
- Achieving and/or maintaining sterility and apyrogenicity

- Use of equipment
- Documentation of the compounding process
- Principles of HEPA-filtered unidirectional airflow within the ISO Class 5 area
- Proper use of primary engineering controls (PECs)
- Principles of movement of materials and personnel within the compounding area

However, the chapter also states that those who compound CSPs or those that have direct oversight over compounding personnel *"must complete training and be able to demonstrate knowledge of principles and competency of skills for performing sterile manipulations and achieving and maintaining appropriate environmental conditions as applicable to their assigned job functions."*[1] This statement leaves staff training needs to be defined by the organization, based on each individual's role. As an example, only those administering a gloved fingertip test need to be trained on media selection, collection technique, and incubation requirements. USP <797> defines oversight as *"the review, monitoring, and supervision of actions taken by personnel, bearing responsibility for those actions, and being available for consultation if and when needed even if not physically present."*[1]

What if you are the only person in the compounding operation?
USP <797> addresses this possibility, requiring that the individual documents that they have received the necessary training and demonstrated competency. This may require the assistance of a consultant or other entity that can provide training and competency evaluation.

Assigned Trainers

Another key element of the training program is those who train and evaluate staff. Training and competency observations may be performed by the designated person(s) or an assigned trainer. An example of an assigned trainer is someone in the organization with extensive knowledge and experience in a certain area, who can train and evaluate others. Another possibility is for the assigned trainer to be an external subject matter expert.

Practical Solution: *Define in your SOPs how a trainer is chosen and what credentials, knowledge base, or experience the individual must have to hold that responsibility. For example, the individual may have a demonstrated mastery of a certain skill set, have specific training in a certain area, or hold a certification. Be sure to identify the assigned trainers in your documentation.*

Training for Those Who Do Not Compound or Oversee Compounding

There may be individuals in an organization who do not compound or oversee compounding, but still hold a vital role in the sterile compounding operation. These individuals still require training but not at the same interval or to the same level as those who compound and oversee compounding. Initial and ongoing training and competency must be defined by facility SOPs for personnel who restock or clean and disinfect the sterile compounding area, perform in-process checks or final verification of CSPs, and only compound immediate-use CSPs.[1] Additionally, the sterile compounding facility can define training and competency requirements for certification providers, contractors, inspectors, surveys, and facility maintenance personnel.

Tables 2 and 3 in USP <797> define the initial and ongoing competency requirements. Table 2 indicates that 4 elements are required for initial training and competency:

1. Garbing and Hand Hygiene Competency
2. Aseptic Manipulation Competency
3. Training and Competency in Maintaining the Quality of the Sterile Compounding Environment
4. Training and Competency in Sterile Compounding Principles and Practices

However, as indicated by Table 3, all are required for ongoing training and competency except for Training and Competency in Maintaining the Quality of the Sterile Compounding Environment. One of the challenges in meeting these requirements is that the chapter only defines requirements for the garbing and hand hygiene and aseptic manipulation competencies, leaving it to each organization to define the other

Exhibit 1
Initial and Ongoing Competencies Defined by USP <797>[1]

Initial Competency Requirements	Ongoing Competency Requirements

Garbing and Hand Hygiene Competency
• 3 times
• Must pass consecutively
• Includes:
  ○ Visual observation
  ○ Gloved fingertip testing
	Garbing and Hand Hygiene Competency
	• 1 time
	• Includes:
	  ○ Visual observation
	  ○ Gloved fingertip testing

Aseptic Manipulation Competency
• Replicates not specified
• Includes:
  ○ Media fill
  ○ Gloved fingertip testing
  ○ Surface Sampling
	Aseptic Manipulation Competency
	• Replicates not specified
	• Includes:
	  ○ Media fill
	  ○ Gloved fingertip testing
	  ○ Surface Sampling

Sterile Compounding Principles and Practices	Sterile Compounding Principles and Practices
Maintaining the quality of the Sterile Compounding Environment	

competencies in their SOPs. Exhibit 1 provides a summary of the specific competencies required by the chapter. Although these are defined in the chapter, remember that training and competency of skills is required for all tasks a compounder or an induvial who oversees compounding performs.

Hand Hygiene and Garbing Competency

There are 2 components to the hand hygiene and garbing competency: a documented visual observation of the hand hygiene and garbing procedure and gloved fingertip sampling. To meet the requirements of the chapter, both activities must be performed initially at least 3 separate times and then at least every 6 months for those compounding Category 1 and 2 CSPs and at least every 3 months for those compounding Category 3 CSPs.

For the observation and sampling, the individual being tested must perform the facility's full hand hygiene and garbing sequence and immediately after donning sterile gloves, without applying sterile 70% IPA, have gloved fingertip samples collected from both hands. It is up to the organization to choose how to document the visual observation. For most organizations a checklist with specific garbing requirements is most effective. The purpose of collecting gloved fingertip samples after fully garbing is to prove the individual is capable of donning sterile gloves without contaminating them.

Exhibit 2 provides a summary of the gloved fingertip sampling that is part of the hand hygiene and garbing competency.

Practical Solution: *The gloved fingertip samples should be collected in the area where the gloves are donned. For example, if the sterile gloves are donned in the buffer room, the samples are collected in the buffer room. If the sterile gloves are donned over the RABS gloves, gloved fingertip samples are collected on the gloves donned inside the RABS. By doing this, you are collecting data most representative of real-life activities.*

Exhibit 2
Overview of Gloved Fingertip Sampling Performed in Conjunction with the Hand Hygiene and Garbing Competency

Purpose	Verify staff can don sterile gloves without contaminating them
Who	Those who compound, have direct oversight of compounding personnel, or as defined by facility SOPs for other staff
When	With the hand hygiene and garbing competency • 3 times initially • Category 1 and 2: at least every 6 months • Category 3: at least every 3 months
Where	Location where gloves are donned
Action Level	>0 CFU per both hands

Follow these steps for collecting, incubating, and analyzing gloved fingertip samples as part of the hand hygiene and garbing competency for those that don sterile gloves in the SEC. Chapter requirements and practical solutions recommendations are indicated.

1.	***Requirement:*** Obtain sampling devices containing TSA with lecithin and polysorbate 80 a. 100 mm settling plates b. 55 mm contact plates c. Paddles
2.	***Requirement:*** Label each sampling device with: a. A personnel identifier b. Right or left hand c. Date and time of sampling
3.	***Practical Solutions Recommendation:*** As soon as the individual finishes donning the sterile gloves, remind them not to touch anything or to apply sterile 70% IPA
4.	***Practical Solutions Recommendation:*** Aseptically open a sampling device and hold it vertically
5.	***Requirement:*** Instruct the individual to roll each fingertip and thumb-tip over the agar surface of the sampling device
6.	***Requirement:*** Close the sample
7.	***Requirement:*** Using a separate sampling device, collect a sample from the other hand
8.	***Requirement:*** Close the sample
9.	***Practical Solutions Recommendation:*** Incubate the sampling devices inverted at 30-35° C for 48 hours to 4 days
10.	***Practical Solutions Recommendation:*** Incubate the sampling devices inverted at 30-35° C for 48 hours to 4 days
11.	***Practical Solutions Recommendation:*** Incubate the sampling devices inverted at 30-35° C for 48 hours to 4 days
12.	***Requirement:*** Read the samples and document the number of recovered CFU on each sample
13.	***Requirement:*** Add together the total number of CFU from both plates
14.	***Requirement:*** Determine whether the CFU count exceeds the action level

When choosing media for gloved fingertip sampling, review the section on Media Selection in Unit 6.

Failure of the hand hygiene and garbing competency is defined as "visual observation of improper hand hygiene and garbing procedures and/or gloved fingertip and thumb sampling results that exceed the action level." The action level for the gloved fingertip samples is a result greater than 0 CFU per both hands. If the staff member fails the competency, it is the responsibility of the sterile compounding organization to determine next steps and identify corrective actions. The competency results and the corrective actions taken because of the failure are documented and maintained as part of the staff member's training record.

You might be wondering why the sample collection device should be held vertically during sample collection? There are 2 reasons for this. First, by holding at this angle there is less of a chance of particulates from the room falling onto the sampling device, resulting in a false positive. Second, by holding the sampling device, you can feel how much pressure the individual is applying to the agar surface. The pressure needs to be enough to transfer microorganisms, but not so hard that the surface of the media is damaged.

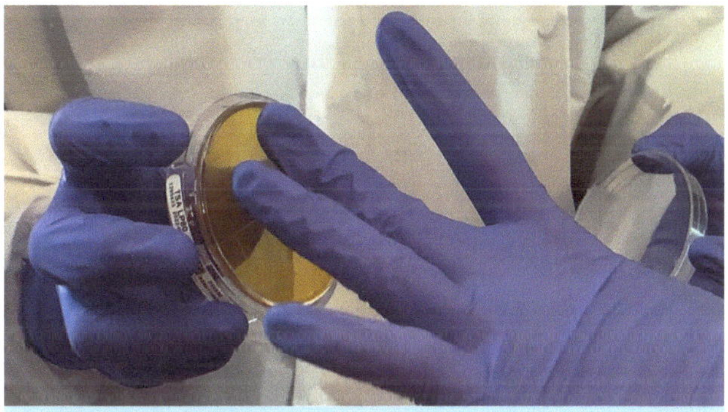

Gloved Fingertip Sampling Reminders

- No sterile 70% IPA before sample collection
- 1 plate per hand
- Rolling motion over the surface
- Sample the pad of the finger/thumb
- Adequate pressure

Photo courtesy of Pure Microbiology, LLC

Practical Solution: *Gloved fingertip sample incubation and analysis considerations - USP <797> does not require gloved fingertip samples to be read after the first incubation as it does for viable air and surface samples. Consider reading the samples and documenting the results after the first incubation. By doing so, any exceeded levels can start to be investigated. As part of the analysis, the chapter does not require that growth on gloved fingertip samples with exceeded action levels be identified. However, in the event of repeated gloved fingertip failures, identification of the organism to the species level provides greater insight into the source and direction to the investigation. These recommendations apply to gloved fingertip sampling performed with both the hand hygiene and garbing and aseptic manipulation competencies.*

Aseptic Manipulation Competency

Regardless of the CSP Category compounded, staff must complete the aseptic manipulation competency, which consists of a media fill test, gloved fingertip sampling, and a surface sample in the DCA. For those who compound Category 1 and 2 CSPs, the competency is required initially and then at least every 6 months. Category 3 compounders are required to complete the competency initially and then at least every 3 months.

Practical Solution: *USP <797> does not specifically require a documented visual observation as part of the aseptic manipulation competency. This is concerning because poor aseptic technique may not always result in a failed competency test. Consideration should be given to developing a written evaluation, which is completed by the person administering the test, to accompany the testing defined in the chapter. By doing so, you will have documentation that the individual has good aseptic technique and follows organization SOPs.*

Media Fill Test

There is no "one size fits all" media fill test, meaning the test will be different for every organization. This is because the chapter requires staff to "simulate the most difficult and challenging compounding procedures and processing conditions" they will encounter, replacing all components with soybean casein digest media.[1] Some organizations will have multiple media fill tests depending on what they compound, and it is the responsibility of the organization to design the testing procedures.

When designing the media fill test, risks to CSP sterility must be identified and included. These include but are not limited to:[1]

- Factors associated with the length of the process that can pose contamination risk
- Number of aseptic additions or transfers
- Number, type, and complexity of manipulations
- Number of personnel in the clean room suite
- Non-sterile-to-sterile compounding procedures
- Container closure types

This chapter guidance is helpful, but it lacks detail and how-to information, especially for those designing media fill tests using equipment like a PN compounder. Fortunately, there is an industry-related document that can fill in some gaps. The Parenteral Drug Association's (PDA) Technical Report 22, titled "Process Simulation for Aseptically Filled Products," discusses principles and concepts as well as specific process simulation considerations. Those with complex compounding processes would benefit from referencing this document when developing their media fill tests.

Did you know that the media fill test required by the chapter is a scaled back version of the process simulation required of aseptic drug manufacturers?

The container used in the compounding process should be what is used in the media fill test. However, there are situations where the container used in compounding would not accommodate the reading of a media fill test. In this case, identical clear containers can be used to aid in the inspection of the container for microbial growth.[3] If this is not possible, it is necessary to transfer the media to a clear container for analysis. The container should be gently shaken, and using aseptic technique, a sufficient volume transferred to a clear container to analyze for microbial growth. This should not be done in a compounding environment in case the media is contaminated.

The media fill test uses soybean-casein digest medium, which is also known as tryptic soy broth. It is a general growth broth that supports a variety or microorganisms, including bacteria and fungi. All microbial growth media is stored according to the manufacturer's instructions and media fill testing must be initiated before the expiration date of the media.

Practical Solutions: *Manufacturers offer a variety of container closure systems filled with sterile soybean-casein digest medium. However, you might not always be able to find what you need, such as syringes filled with media to include on a PN compounder. If this is the case, containers of media can be prepared aseptically in 2 different ways. One way would be to include the preparation of these containers as part of the media fill test. The other way would be to aseptically prepare the containers a few days before the test and pre-incubate them at 20-25° C for at least 48 hours and inspect for microbial growth before use.*

Those who perform sterile-to-sterile compounding can either purchase commercially prepared sterile media in its final form or prepare their own media starting from non-sterile powder. For the commercially prepared media, the chapter requires that a certificate of analysis (COA) be obtained stating that the lot will support the growth of microorganisms. However, even those preparing their own soybean-casein digest medium from powder should have a COA on file. Additionally, the chapter does require that those preparing their own media for a sterile-to-sterile media fill perform growth promotion testing for each batch prepared, as described in USP General Chapter Sterility Tests <71>. This requires laboratory capabilities and is not something a sterile compounding organization can perform. When performing a media fill test simulating sterile-to-sterile compounding, sterile water or sterile saline cannot be introduced into the process, unless the media manufacturer specifies this is necessary. Diluting the media could prevent it from supporting microbial growth, resulting in false negatives.

For those simulating non-sterile-to-sterile compounding, the media is prepared by dissolving commercially available non-sterile soybean–casein digest powder in non-bacteriostatic water to make a 3% non-sterile solution. The media manufacturer will also provide instructions for the media preparation. Follow the manufacturer's instructions for preparation if they result in a percent solution other than 3%. This media is then used as the components in the non-sterile-to-sterile compounding process. Since the media is being prepared by the sterile compounding organization, it is important to prepare at least 1 container that will serve as a positive control, showing that the media can support growth. To do this, prior to the sterilization step, transfer prepared media to the final container closure system. Incubate with the

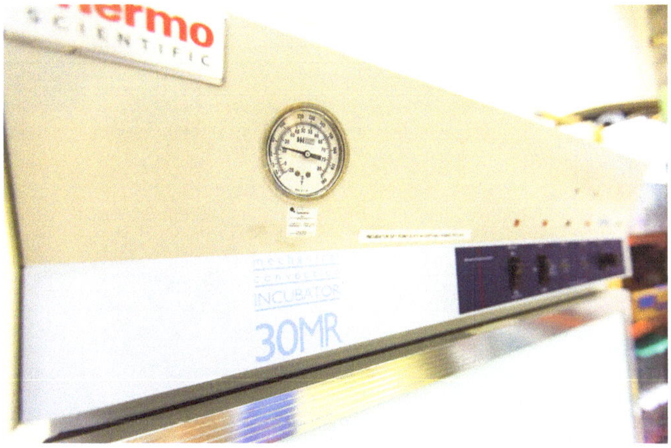

Photo courtesy of Contec, Inc.

media fill test samples. During analysis, look for visible turbidity in the final container. If the positive control does not exhibit turbidity or other microbial growth patterns, the media fill test utilizing that same lot of media is not valid.

Media fill test samples are incubated, in an incubator for 7 days at 20-25° C and 7 days at 30-35° C. Incubation may start at either temperature. It is critical that the test samples are incubated for 14 days. This is because at least 1 million bacteria per milliliter of broth are needed for turbidity to be detected with the unaided eye and some microorganisms need more time to grow than others.[4] Therefore, a media fill test sample that appears clear on day 3 of incubation may be contaminated and not appear turbid until day 7 or even up until day 14. Any visible turbidity or other visual manifestations of growth in the media in any of the container closure unit(s) on or before the end of the incubation period is considered a media fill test failure.

Practical Solution: *Pre- and Post-Incubation Media Fill Sample Inspection – USP <797> does not provide detail on media fill inspection activities, but this information can be found in PDA's Technical Report 22. Prior to placing samples in the incubator, they should be inverted and swirled to be sure the media contacts all internal surfaces.*[3] *This is especially important for vials that are aseptically filled and then stoppered/crimped, as the stopper could become contaminated but never contact the media. Prior to incubation, samples should also be inspected for cracks, improper closures, or another defect that could affect the sterility of the container.*[3] *Post-incubation inspection should be performed by trained staff who are familiar with the different microbial growth patterns that can occur in a broth.*

Exhibit 3

Microbial Growth Pattern in Soybean-Casein Digest Medium

Gloved Fingertip Sampling After the Media Fill

As part of the aseptic manipulation competency, gloved fingertip samples are collected after the completion of the media fill test. This sample collection occurs inside the PEC, whether an LAFW, BSC, or RABS. Gloves are not to be sprayed with sterile 70% IPA immediately prior to the sample collection.

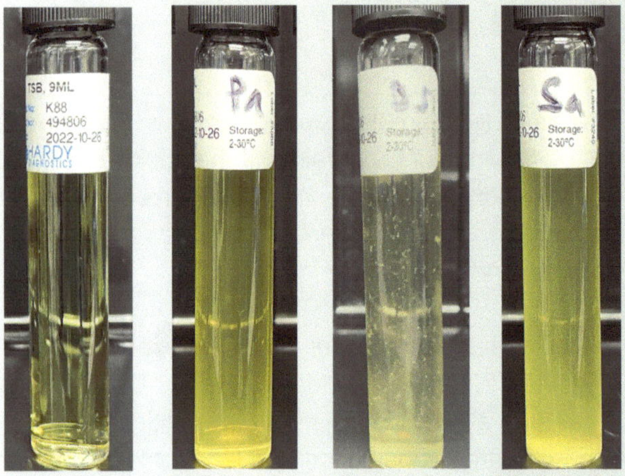

Clear | Turbid | Flocculent | Sediment

Purpose	Verify staff can keep the microbial bioburden on their gloves low during a compounding activity
Who	Those who compound or have direct oversight of compounding personnel
When	With the aseptic manipulation competency Initially • Category 1 and 2: at least every 6 months • Category 3: at least every 3 months
Where	In the PEC
Action Level	>3 CFU per both hands

Those reading the media fill test samples must be able to recognize different microbial growth patterns in media. Some microorganisms will render the media uniformly turbid. Others will settle to the bottom of the container, forming a sediment. Flocculent growth may also be seen, which can look like flakes or chunks in the broth. Exhibit 3 provides a visual comparison of these different growth patterns.

Follow these steps for collecting, incubating, and analyzing gloved fingertip samples that are part of the aseptic manipulation competency. Chapter requirements and practical solutions are indicated.

1.	***Requirement:*** Obtain sampling devices containing TSA with lecithin and polysorbate 80 a. 100 mm settling plates b. 55 mm contact plates c. Paddles
2.	***Requirement:*** Place them in the PEC
3.	***Practical Solutions Recommendation:*** As soon as the individual finishes the media fill test, remind them not to touch anything or to apply sterile 70% IPA
4.	***Practical Solutions Recommendation:*** Aseptically open a sampling device, leaving it on the PEC work surface if it is a plate
5.	***Requirement:*** Instruct the individual to roll each fingertip and thumb-tip over the agar surface of the sampling device
6.	***Requirement:*** Close the sample (remove and discard sampled gloves and don new gloves)
7.	***Requirement:*** Using a separate sampling device, collect a sample from the other hand
8.	***Requirement:*** Close the sample
9.	***Requirement:*** Remove the samples from the PEC
10.	***Requirement:*** Label each sampling device with: a. A personnel identifier b. Right or left hand c. Date and time of sampling
11.	***Practical Solutions Recommendation:*** Incubate the sampling devices inverted at 30-35° C for 48 hours to 4 days
12.	***Practical Solutions Recommendation:*** Read the samples and document the number of recovered colony forming units (CFU) on each sample
13.	***Requirement:*** Incubate the sampling devices inverted at 20-25° C for 5-7 days
14.	***Practical Solutions Recommendation:*** Read the samples and document the number of recovered CFU on each sample
15.	***Requirement:*** Add together the total number of CFU from both plates
16.	***Requirement:*** Determine whether the CFU count exceeds the action level

Failure of the gloved fingertip samples collected with the media fill is defined as a result greater than the action level 3 CFU per both hands.

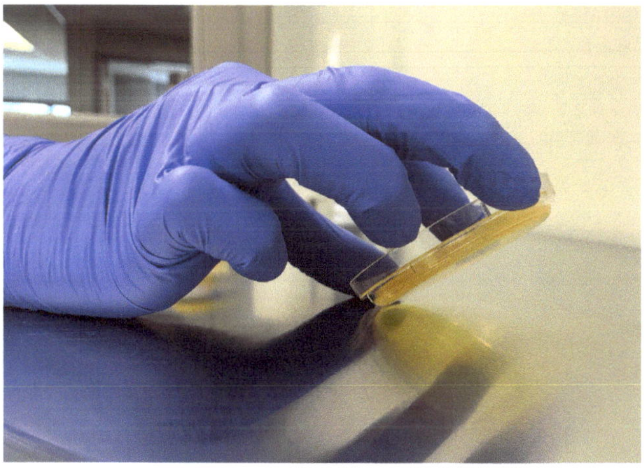

Photo courtesy of Pure Microbiology, LLC

Surface Sampling After the Media Fill

The collection of the surface sample in the DCA after the media fill test is done as defined in Unit 6 Viable Air and Surface Sampling. Be sure this sample is collected before the area is sanitized with sterile 70% IPA or cleaned and disinfected. The PEC action levels defined in Unit 6 apply to this sample. Additionally, if the number of CFUs recovered exceeds the action level, the growth must be identified to at least the genus level.

Aseptic Manipulation Competency Failure

If a staff member fails any portion of the aseptic manipulation competency, it is considered an overall failure. It is the responsibility of the sterile compounding organization to determine appropriate corrective actions, which could include additional training, increased supervision during compounding until successful completion of the competency, or removal from compounding. The individual is required to repeat the competency evaluation. The sterile compounding organization must define the appropriate timeframe between attempts of the competency evaluation. Competency results and any corrective actions taken to remediate the staff member's aseptic technique are documented and maintained as part of their training record.

Training and Competency Documentation

As was previously mentioned, USP <797> requires documentation of the training and competency evaluations. This documentation could be paper-based or through an electronic means. For training, be sure to capture at least the trainer and trainee names, topics covered, date, and clear indication of training completion.

USP <797> defines information that must be captured as part of the competency documentation. At a minimum documentation must include:[1]

1. Name of person evaluated
2. Name or identification of the evaluator
3. Evaluation date and time
4. Media and components used, including manufacturer
5. Expiration date and lot number for any items used
6. Starting temperature for each interval of incubation
7. Dates of incubation
8. Results
9. Name of identification of individual reading and documenting the results

Practical Solution: *Document the time of incubation – The chapter does not require the documentation of the time samples are placed into the incubator, only the date. Consider including the time the samples went into and came out of the incubator. This is especially important for samples that have a minimum incubation time of 48 hours. As an example, if samples start incubation at 4:00 pm on Tuesday, they cannot be read until 4:00 pm on Thursday. If only the incubation date is documented, the individual reading the samples will not know what time to perform the analysis, and this could result in an incubation period of less than 48 hours.*

Exhibit 4

Testing Required for the USP <797> Defined Competencies

Initial Competencies	Subsequent Competencies
Visual observation of hand hygiene and garbing (3 times)	Visual observation of hand hygiene and garbing (1 time)
Gloved fingertip sampling post-hand hygiene and garbing (3 times)	Gloved fingertip sampling post-hand hygiene and garbing (1 time)
Media fill test	Media fill test
Gloved fingertip sampling post-media fill test	Gloved fingertip sampling post-media fill test
Surface sample in the DCA post-media fill test	Surface sample in the DCA post-media fill test

Summary

The development of robust training and implementation of valuable competency evaluations can fundamentally change an organization. Staff equipped with the knowledge and skill to perform their assigned tasks will be more engaged in workflow and process improvement of the compounding operation. On the other side of that, "no amount of managerial oversight can make up for staff that has not been adequately trained."[2] While the chapter does define 2 required competencies, as summarized in Exhibit 4, additional competencies will need to be developed based on operations and assigned tasks.

References

1. United States Pharmacopeia. <797> Pharmaceutical Compounding—Sterile Preparations. Revision. November 2022.
2. Douglass, K. Cleanrooms & Compounding: Staff Training. *Pharmacy Purchasing & Products.* October 2007. Vol. 4 No. 10.
3. Parental Drug Association. Technical Report 22 Process Simulation for Aseptically Filled Products. 2011.
4. Tille PM. *Bailey and Scott's Diagnostic Microbiology* 14th ed. Page 87. 2014.

UNIT 8

Summary: Training and Evaluation Summary

Training and competency frequencies are defined by USP <797>. This table summarizes those requirements.

Initial training and qualification by demonstrating knowledge and competency in tasks defined by role	
Demonstration of competency and testing in required areas at least every 12 months	
Visual observation of hand hygiene and garbing 3 times initially	
Gloved fingertip sampling post-hand hygiene and garbing 3 times initially	
Media fill test	
Gloved fingertip sampling post-media fill test	
Surface sample in the DCA post-media fill test	
Those compounding Category 1 and 2 CSPs perform the following every 6 months:	**Those compounding Category 3 CSPs perform the following every 3 months:**
Visual observation of hand hygiene and garbing	
Gloved fingertip sampling post-hand hygiene and garbing	
Media fill test	
Gloved fingertip sampling post media fill test	
Surface sample in the DCA post media fill test	

The following is a general gloved fingertip sample collection, incubation, and analysis procedure. When collecting samples with the aseptic manipulation competency, be sure the sample collection is performed in the PEC.

1. Obtain sampling devices containing TSA with lecithin and polysorbate 80
    a. 100 mm settling plates
    b. 55 mm contact plates
    c. Paddles
2. Remind individual not to apply sterile 70% IPA to gloves
3. Aseptically open a sampling device
4. Instruct the individual to roll each fingertip and thumb-tip over the agar surface of the sampling device
5. Close the sample
6. Using a separate sampling device collect a sample from the other hand
7. Close the sample
8. Label each sampling device with:
    a. A personnel identifier
    b. Right or left hand
    c. Date and time of sampling
    9. Incubate the sampling devices inverted at 30-35° C for 48-72 hours
10. Read the samples and document the number of recovered colony forming units (CFU) on each sample
11. Incubate the sampling devices inverted at 20-25° C for 5-7 days
12. Read the samples and document the number of recovered CFU on each sample
13. Add together the total number of CFU from both plates
14. Determine whether the CFU count exceeds the action level

UNIT 9

Standard Operating Procedures (SOPs) and Other Documentation

Quality is a simple term that can have very different meanings depending on the services or products a company or organization provides. USP General Chapter <797> provides quality-related requirements for sterile compounding organizations. However, these are minimum requirements, and to have an effective quality program, additional processes and procedures must be incorporated. In this unit we'll explore minimum chapter requirements, as well as practical solutions to meet and exceed compliance.

What Is Quality?

Take a moment to think about how you define quality. Maybe you associate quality with a product being made right or meeting expectations. If so, you are not too far off from the American Society for Quality (ASQ) definition. According to ASQ, quality is a subjective term, where each industry may have its own definition. But in its simplest form, quality can be defined 2 ways:[1]

1. The characteristics of a product or service that bear on its ability to meet stated or implied needs
2. A product or service free from deficiencies

Both definitions apply to sterile compounding. For the first definition, the CSP must have the intended effect, meeting the patient's therapeutic need. For the second definition, we can think of being "free of deficiencies" as being free from particulate and microbial contamination.

Quality-Related Definitions

Being familiar with quality-related terms can clarify why an organization is set up and operates in a specific way. First, let's define quality management and quality management system. Quality management is *"managing activities and resources of an organization to achieve objectives and prevent non-conformances."*[1] In a sterile compounding organization this is the management of everything done to ensure safe, efficacious medications. The quality management system (QMS) is the *"formal system that documents the structure, processes, roles, responsibilities and procedures required to achieve effective quality management."*[1] This would be the SOPs, assigned roles, and designated workflows. We'll explore the QMS in more detail later in the unit.

Quality Management System (QMS) Principles

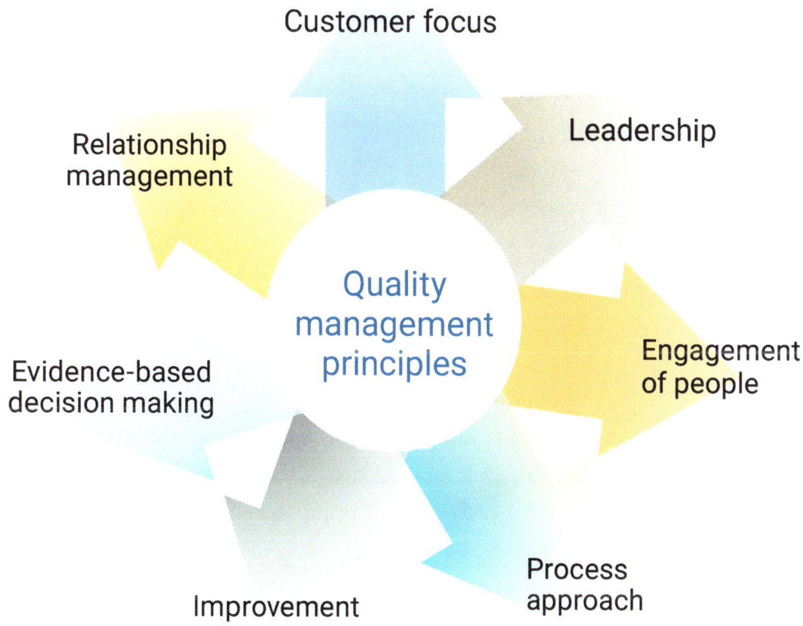
Customer focus
Leadership
Engagement of people
Process approach
Improvement
Evidence-based decision making
Relationship management
Quality management principles

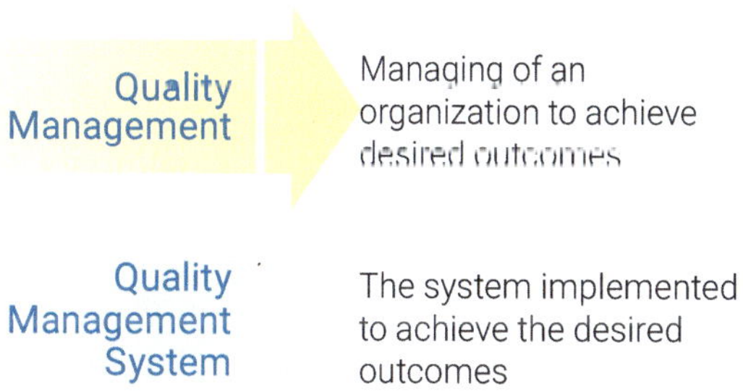

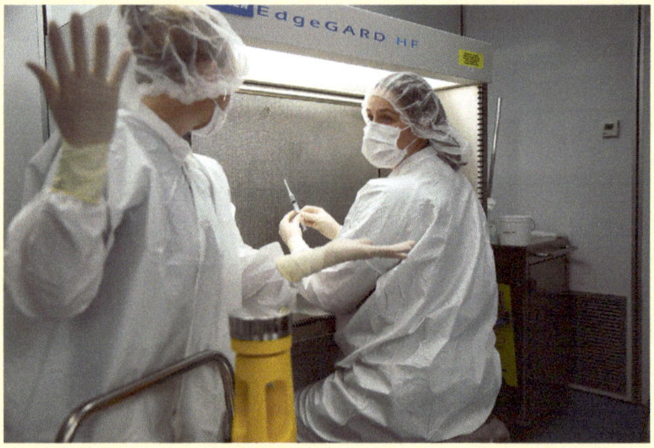

As famous quality guru W. Edwards Deming said, "Quality is everyone's responsibility."[3] USP <797> defines numerous quality-related responsibilities of the designated person, but it also defines 1 very crucial staff responsibility. Staff must recognize actual or potential problems, deviations, failures, or errors that could negatively impact the quality of a CSP and report them to the designated person.[2] These could include issues with equipment, the clean room, materials, personnel, the compounding process, or testing. Reporting potential issues is just as important as reporting actual issues. Bringing an issue to light before there is an actual problem could be invaluable to a patient and the organization.

Photo courtesy of Contec, Inc.

There are 2 other very important terms—quality assurance and quality control—that are sometimes used interchangeably but are different. Exhibit 1 provides a comparison of the ASQ and USP <797> definitions.

Quality Management System (QMS)

In simple terms, the QMS can be defined as the system implemented to achieve the desired outcomes. When we look at USP <797>, it could be seen as a loose framework for a QMS, requiring the sterile compounding organization to add the details specific to its own operation. USP <797> does not use the term QMS but does indicate the need for QA and QC programs. Based on the chapter there must be written QA and QC programs that establish a system of:[2]

1. Adherence to procedures
2. Prevention and detection of errors and other quality problems
3. Evaluation of complaints and adverse events
4. Appropriate investigations and corrective actions

The chapter also references USP General Chapter <1163> Quality Assurance in Sterile Compounding. This informational chapter describes the 9 minimum components of a quality assurance program, which include:[4]

1. Training
2. Standard operating procedures
3. Documentation
4. Verification

Exhibit 1

Comparison of ASQ and USP <797> and Quality Definitions[1,2]

	ASQ Definition	USP <797> Definition	Take Away
Quality Assurance (QA)	All the planned and systematic activities implemented within the quality system that can be demonstrated to provide confidence that a product or service will fulfill requirements for quality	A system of procedures, activities, and oversight that ensures that the compounding process consistently meets quality standards	• Have a defined system • Comply with applicable standards and guidance • Define what quality means for your CSPs
Quality Control (QC)	The operational techniques and activities used to fulfill requirements for quality	The sampling, testing, and documentation of results that, taken together, ensure that specifications have been met before release of the CSP	• Identify a process for confirming CSP quality • Confirm CSPs meet quality requirements before use

5. Testing
6. Cleaning, disinfecting, and safety
7. Containers, packaging, repackaging, labeling, and storage
8. Outsourcing
9. Responsible personnel

All the items covered in the 2 USP chapters are important parts of a QMS, but the true quality elements are not clearly defined. ASQ provides the elements of a quality management system, which include:[5]

1. Quality manual, policy, and objectives
2. Procedures, instructions, and records
3. Data management
4. Internal processes
5. Customer satisfaction
6. Improvement opportunities
7. Quality analysis

For this unit, the term QMS will be used as it truly encompasses everything that is expected of a sterile compounding organization regarding quality expectations.

When we look at the USP and ASQ elements, there is definite overlap, but the ASQ elements are a bit broader, allowing for the inclusion of more quality-related concepts that are not specifically defined in the USP chapters. Exhibit 2 lists the high-level QMS elements and the associated USP and quality elements that would create a comprehensive QMS for a sterile compounding organization.

Sterile compounding operations that are part of a larger organization may already have a robust QMS, where the overarching quality concepts, such as document control and vendor management, may be defined. However, smaller independent companies are responsible for developing the entire QMS.

> **To learn more about QMS elements,** such as corrective and preventive actions (CAPA), change control, and auditing, visit asq.org.

Benefits of a QMS

The 2 main benefits of implementing a QMS are meeting the customer's requirements and meeting the organization's requirements.[5] Meeting the customer's requirements builds confidence that your organization can meet their needs, which builds a positive reputation, leading to more customers, sales, and business. The biggest organization requirement is regulatory compliance. Consistently meeting regulatory compliance is necessary for continued operations. Additional advantages of a well-functioning QMS include:[5]

- Process definition, improvement, and control
- Waste reduction
- Mistake prevention
- Low costs
- Facilitation and identification of training opportunities
- Staff engagement

Exhibit 2

High-Level QMS Elements and the Associated Sterile Compounding Quality Elements

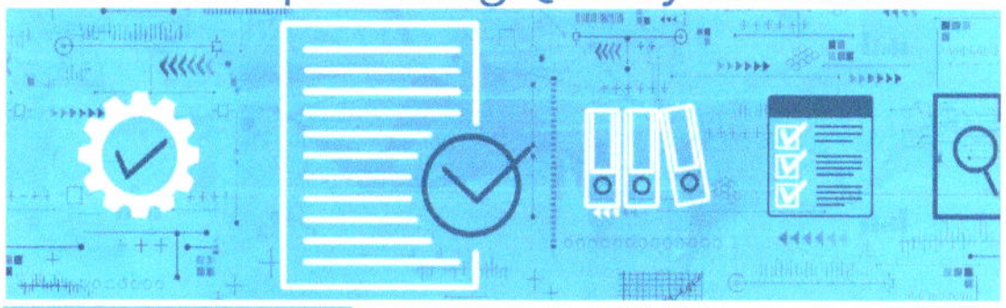

QMS element	Associated quality elements
Quality manual, policy, and objectives	Regulatory compliance
Procedures, instructions, and records	• SOPs • Master formulation records • Compounding records • Training records • Logs
Data management	• Storage of paper-based documention • Workflow managment system • Record access
Internal processes	• Training • Defined workflows • Document control • Change control • Process control • Designated responsibilities • Vendor management • Receipt of materials • Facility maintenance
Customer satisfaction	• Complaint handling • Adverse events management • Recalls
Improvement opportunities	• Corrective and preventive action (CAPA) • Internal audits • External audits
Quality analysis	• Stability testing • Release testing • Viable sampling

What is an internal system audit?

Let's break the internal system audit down into its components. An internal audit is performed within an organization, by employees. It is also known as a first-party audit. The goal is to identify the organization's strengths and weaknesses in comparison to its own procedures and regulatory requirements.[6] Essentially, it examines if the organization is following its own SOPs and meeting regulations. A system audit is a documented activity that verifies elements of the system are appropriate and effective and have been implemented according to specific requirements. This goes beyond just meeting regulatory requirements and requires an evaluation of effectiveness. Therefore, an internal system audit of the QMS reviews conformance to SOPs, contract commitments, and regulatory requirements—and assesses the effectiveness of the system.[6]

QMS Requirements

For USP <797> chapter compliance, SOPs must describe the roles, duties, and training of those responsible for each aspect of the QMS. At least once every 12 months, the overall QMS must be reviewed by the designated person(s). During the review any issues are noted, the findings are documented, and appropriate action must be taken, if required. When we compare these chapter requirements to quality activities, they are essentially an internal system audit and the CAPA process.

Quality Assurance and Quality Control in the QMS

Within the overall QMS there are quality assurance (QA) procedures and quality control (QC) activities. Remember, QA is the set of procedures used to ensure quality, while QC is the testing used to prove that quality. USP <797> includes numerous QA and QC components, although you won't find them all under the quality section of the chapter because the chapter is essentially a quality system. In the rest of the unit, we will review some of the quality-related chapter elements listed in Exhibit 3.

Documentation and Document Control

USP <797> describes requirements for what documents need to exist, how information is recorded, and how the documents need to be maintained. These requirements apply to all facilities where CSPs are prepared. To be compliant with USP <797>, an organization must:[2]

1. Maintain written or electronic documentation to demonstrate chapter compliance
2. Comply with all laws and regulations of the applicable regulatory jurisdiction
3. Document in a legible manner
4. Store documentation in a manner to prevent deterioration or loss
5. Maintain all required compounding records for a particular CSP for at least 2 years after preparation or as required by applicable regulatory jurisdiction, whichever is longer

As mentioned, the chapter requires documentation to demonstrate compliance. USP <797> provides a list of the required documentation in Section 20; however, it does not include some of the other documentation requirements from other sections of the chapter. The Section 20 requirements include:[2]

- Personnel training, competency assessments, and qualification records
- Certification reports
- Environmental air and surface monitoring procedures and results
- Equipment records, including calibration, verification, and maintenance reports
- Receipt of components

Exhibit 3

USP <797> Quality-Related Elements

Quality Assurance	Quality Control
• Documentation and document control • SOPs • Master formulation and compounding records • Labeling • Notification of out-of-specification CSPs • Recalls • Handling complaints and adverse events • Training • Hand hygiene and garbing • Facilities and engineering controls • Cleaning and disinfection • Work practices • Establishing BUDs • Sterilization and depyrogenation	• Visual inspection • Stability testing • Sterility testing • Bacterial endotoxin testing • Potency testing • pH testing • Filter integrity testing • Personnel competencies • Certification of engineering controls • Temperature and humidity monitoring • Viable air and surface sampling • Use of biological, endotoxin, and physicochemical indicators

- SOPs
- Master formulation records and compounding records, if required
- Release inspection and testing records
- Information related to complaints and adverse events including corrective actions
- Results of any investigations, including training, certification, viable sampling failures, and the associated corrective actions

Keep in mind that this list is not all inclusive and other documents may be necessary to fully demonstrate chapter compliance.

Practical Solution: *Implementing a Successful Document Control System - USP <797> does not provide guidance on managing and controlling documents, leaving it to the organization to implement a system. To have a successful and robust system be sure to include procedures for documents, including:*

- *Identification, such as document type and a numbering system*
- *Version control*
- *Access*
- *Filing*
- *Storage, maintenance, and disposal*

In addition, include documentation practices, especially if you have a partial or full paper-based system. Good documentation practices are based on the acronym ALCOA, which stands for attributable, legible, contemporaneously recorded, original, and accurate.[7]

SOPs

SOPs documenting the compounding process and other support activities are required by USP <797> for any facility that prepares CSPs. This means there should be an SOP for nearly everything that occurs in the organization related to sterile compounding. Additionally, the categories of CSPs compounded by the organization must be defined in the SOPs.

The designated person has several SOP-related responsibilities, which include:

- Ensuring that SOPs are appropriate and implemented
- Taking corrective actions if problems, deviations, failures, or errors associated with organizational SOPs are identified
- Confirming that all personnel who perform or oversee compounding or support activities are trained in the SOPs
- Reviewing SOPs at least every 12 months and documenting the review
- Overseeing changes to an SOP
- Communicating SOP revisions to appropriate personnel

SOPs are important because they document the process that must be followed, ensuring consistency in how activities are performed and ideally eliminating human error. However, many times SOPs do not have sufficient detail to ensure consistency among staff members. Let's look at a hand hygiene procedure for a sterile compounding facility.

1. Remove a nail pick from the container.
2. Wet hands, apply soap, and lather.
3. Use the nail pick to clean under nails.
4. Apply soap and lather fingers to elbows for 30 seconds.
5. Thoroughly rinse hands and forearms.
6. Dry hands and forearms with a low-lint wipe.

Does the procedure have enough detail? Are all the steps clearly defined to ensure consistency among staff? Not likely. Let's now look at a hand hygiene procedure with sufficient detail and clear steps.

1. Remove a disposable nail pick from the container and set it on the edge of the sink.
2. Wet hands and arms to the elbow using warm water.
3. Slightly lather hands with Brand X soap.
4. Under warm running water, use the disposable nail pick to clean each nail.
5. Dispose of the nail pick in the trash can next to the sink.
6. Apply additional soap if needed, and lather from the fingertips to the elbows for at least 30 seconds, tracking time on the clock above the sink.
7. Thoroughly rinse hands and forearms with warm water, being sure all soap has been removed.
8. Gently shake excess water from hands and forearms while over the sink.
9. Dry hands and forearms thoroughly with disposable, low-lint wipers.
10. Dispose of the wipers in the trash can next to the sink.

These steps are much clearer and sets the expectations for the process. To make this version of the SOP even better, consider adding pictures of each step.

Master Formulation Records and Compounding Records

A master formulation record (MFR) is the "recipe" for preparing a CSP. It details how the CSP is to be prepared. A compounding record documents the actual preparation of the CSP or the repackaging process. USP <797> requires an MFR be created for all CSPs prepared from non-sterile ingredient(s) or CSPs prepared for more than 1 patient, while a CR must be created for all Category 1, Category 2, and Category 3 CSPs and immediate-use CSPs prepared for more than 1 patient.[2]

Because a change to an MFR could significantly alter efficacy and safety of a CSP, any alterations must be approved and documented. The following information must be included in an MFR:[2]

- Name, strength or activity, and dosage form of the CSP
- Identities and amounts of all ingredients
- Type and size of container closure system(s)
- Complete instructions for preparing the CSP
  - Equipment
  - Supplies
  - Compounding steps
  - Special precautions
- Physical description of the final CSP
- BUD and storage requirements
- Reference source to support the stability of the CSP
- QC procedures
- Any other information needed to describe the compounding process

***Practical Solution:** MFRs for All CSPs Prepared – The goal of the MFR is to ensure consistency and repeatability in the compounding process. Home infusion providers need to reduce practice variation through SOPs and the use of MFRs.[7] Even if the organization does not compound CSPs that require MFRs, consider having 1 for every formulation.*

A compounding record can take a variety of formats. It could be a defined document that is completed during compounding, a prescription or medication order, or a label. It could even be multiple documents combined to act as the compounding record. Any format is acceptable if all the required information, as listed below, is retrievable.[2]

- Name, strength or activity, and dosage form of the CSP
- Date and time of preparation of the CSP
- Assigned internal identification number such as a prescription, order, or lot number
- Identification of individuals involved in the compounding process

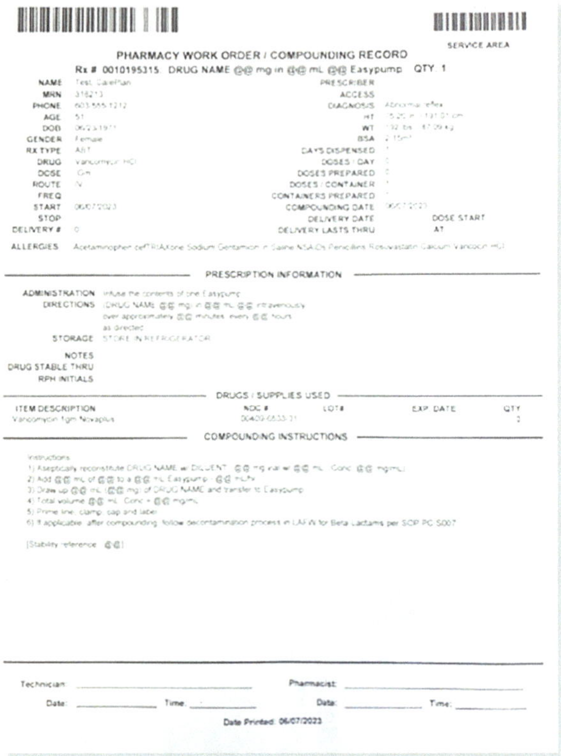
SERVICE AREA

PHARMACY WORK ORDER / COMPOUNDING RECORD

Rx # 0010195315 DRUG NAME @@ mg in @@ mL @@ Easypump QTY: 1

NAME / MRN / PHONE / AGE / DOB / GENDER / RX TYPE / DRUG / DOSE / ROUTE / FREQ / START / STOP / DELIVERY #

PRESCRIBER / ACCESS / DIAGNOSIS / HT / WT / BSA / DAYS DISPENSED / DOSES / DAY / DOSES PREPARED / DOSES / CONTAINER / CONTAINERS PREPARED / COMPOUNDING DATE / DELIVERY DATE / DELIVERY LASTS THRU / DOSE START / AT

ALLERGIES

PRESCRIPTION INFORMATION

ADMINISTRATION DIRECTIONS

STORAGE

NOTES

DRUG STABLE THRU

RPH INITIALS

DRUGS / SUPPLIES USED

ITEM DESCRIPTION	NDC #	LOT#	EXP. DATE	QTY

COMPOUNDING INSTRUCTIONS

Technician: ______ Pharmacist: ______

Date: ______ Time: ______ Date: ______ Time: ______

Date Printed: 06/07/2023

Sample courtesy of New England Life Care

- Identification of individuals verifying the final CSP
- Component information
  - Name of each component
  - Vendor
  - Lot number
  - Expiration date
  - Weight or volume
  - Strength or activity
- Total quantity compounded
- Final yield
- Assigned BUD and storage requirements
- Results of QC procedures
- If applicable, the compounding record must also include:
  - MFR reference for the CSP
  - Calculations for the determination and verification of quantities and/or concentrations of components

Not sure what to include in the compounding record? Use the MFR as the basis for the compounding record. Just add spaces for recording the information needed to complete the compounding record.

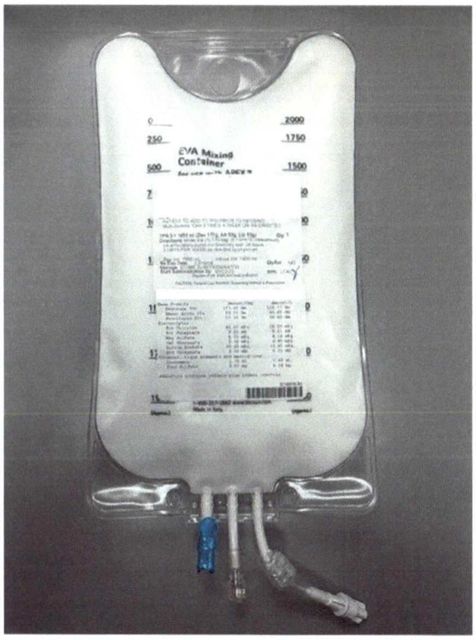

Photo courtesy of New England Life Care

A properly labeled PN

Exhibit 4

CSP Label and Labeling Requirements

Label on Each CSP Container	Labeling
• Assigned internal identification number • Active ingredients and their amounts, activity, or concentration • Storage conditions if other than controlled room temperature • BUD • Dosage form • Total amount or volume if it is not obvious from the container • If it is a single-dose container, a statement stating such when space permits • If it is a multiple-dose container, a statement stating such	• Route of administration • Any special handling instructions • Any warning statements • Contact information of the compounding facility if the CSP is to be sent outside of the facility or health care system in which it was compounded • SHOULD – indication the preparation is compounded

Labeling

USP <797> references USP <7> Labeling for label-related definitions. Labeling designates "all labels and other written, printed, or graphic matter on an article's immediate container or on, or in, any package or wrapper in which it is enclosed, except any outer shipping container."[9] Label refers to the part of the labeling on the immediate container.[9] It is important to understand the difference so you can ensure the right information is displayed in the right place.

Proper labeling prevents errors during storage, dispensing, and use. All CSPs, except those prepared under the immediate-use provision, must be labeled with appropriate, legible identifying information. Although USP <797> provides labeling requirements, the organization may fall under the jurisdiction of other regulatory bodies that will require compliance with their labeling laws and regulations. Be sure to review all applicable requirements when determining the information that will be included on the labels. Exhibit 4 indicates the minimum required CSP container label information and labeling that must be displayed on the CSP.

Each sterile compounding organization must develop labeling procedures to prevent labeling errors and CSP mix-ups. It is critical that SOPs dictate a clear process that is followed by all. There must also be a process for verifying the label to ensure it conforms with the prescription or medication order, the MFR, if required, and the compounding record, if required.

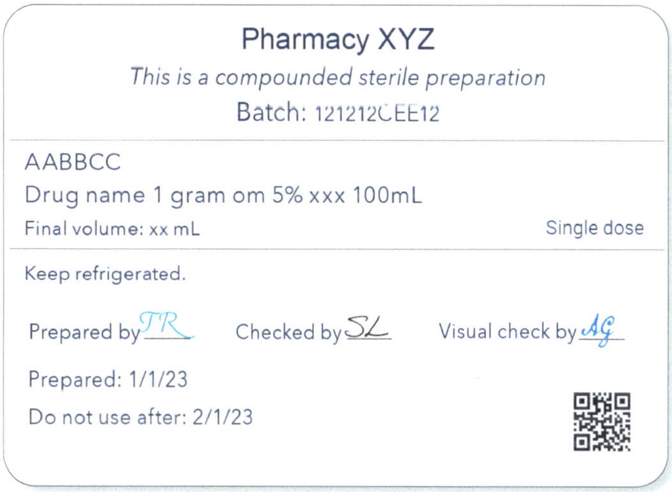

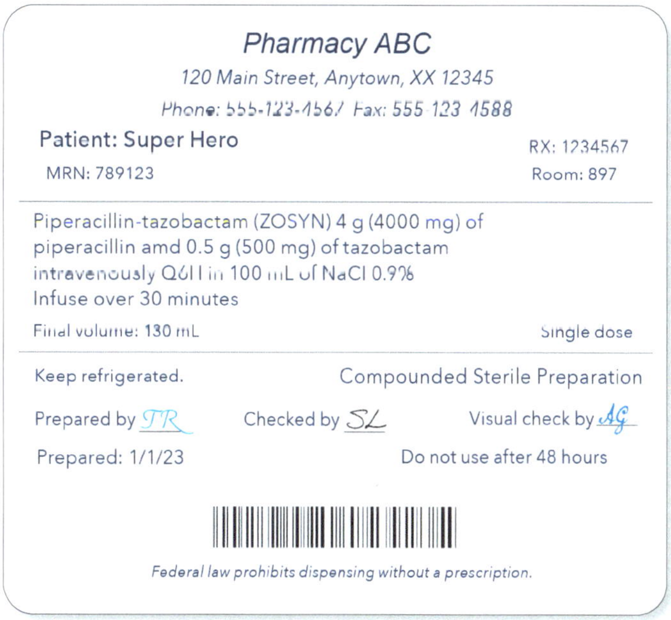

Notification of Out-of-Specification and Recalls

As part of a robust QMS, there must be SOPs in place describing how to handle dispensed CSPs that do not meet specifications and issue a recall. The hope is that these SOPs are never used.

There may be an instance where a CSP needs to be dispensed or administered before the results of release testing are known. A common example of this is administering a CSP prior to sterility testing being complete. If this is a possibility for the sterile compounding organization, it must have procedures in place to notify the prescriber, recall the medication, quarantine remaining stock, and perform an investigation. Exhibit 5 describes considerations for each of these requirements.

Exhibit 5

Steps for Notification About and Recall of Out-of-Specification Dispensed CSPs

Notify the prescriber

Indicate the type of failure and how it could cause patient harm

Recall the medication

This includes unused dispensed CSPs

Quarantine remaining stock

Clearly segrate the CSPs in question from acceptable CSPs

Investigate

Determine if other lots are affected and recall if necessary

USP <797> defines the essential components of a recall SOP. The SOP must contain procedures to:[2]

- Determine the severity of the problem and the urgency for implementation and completion of the recall
- Determine the distribution of any affected CSP, including the date and quantity of distribution
- Identify patients who have received the CSP
- Dispose of the recalled CSP and how to document the disposal
- Investigate and document the reason for failure

Any time a recall is initiated, the sterile compounding facility must document the occurrence. All actions taken in association with the recall should be documented in a comprehensive investigation and the root cause of the investigation should be addressed as part of a CAPA program. The goal is to prevent the issue from recurring. USP <797> also requires that the recall "be reported to appropriate regulatory bodies as required by laws and regulations of the applicable regulatory jurisdiction."[2] Each sterile compounding organization must identify the reporting requirements for their location.

Handling Complaints

Any business may receive a complaint, even a sterile compounding organization. It's important to have an SOP that provides a consistent process for receiving, documenting, researching, and analyzing complaints, enabling a measurable continuous improvement process. And, ultimately, improving service delivery and patient outcomes.

The most common ways complaints are received are in person, over the phone, through an email, or via letter. However, complaints could also come through customer surveys or indirectly through a state department of health, board of pharmacy, or the U.S. Food and Drug Administration (FDA).

All these possible submission options should be considered when developing the complaint handling process, to ensure the complaint quickly reaches the designated person.

Complaints could include issues with quality, labeling, or possible adverse reactions related to a specific CSP. Each complaint must be evaluated by the designated person to determine if there is a potential quality problem with the CSP. There is the possibility that a complaint may not require any further investigation. However, any complaint deemed to be due to CSP quality is thoroughly investigated and appropriate corrective actions are identified. As part of the investigation, determine if the quality problem affects other CSPs, and apply the identified corrective actions to the potentially affected CSPs as well. Consider whether to initiate a recall of potentially affected CSPs and whether to cease sterile compounding operations until the implemented corrective actions have been deemed effective.

The documentation associated with a complaint includes the details of the complaint and the completed investigation. When a complaint is received, a written or electronic record is completed, capturing relevant information. The information collected will be determined by your organization. Exhibit 6 lists chapter-related and recommended information elements.

Exhibit 6

Information to Include in a Complaint Record

Chapter Information	Recommended Information
MUST • Name or identifier of the complainant • Date the complaint was received • Nature of the complaint • Response to the complaint SHOULD • Name of the CSP • Strength of the CSP • CSP assigned internal identification	• Contact information of the complainant • Role of the person making the complaint (e.g. physician, nurse, materials management personnel) • Name of the designated person notified • Date designated person notified • Name of person who received the complaint

All complaint records, including the investigation, must be readily retrievable and maintained by the sterile compounding organization. Any CSP returned in connection with a complaint is quarantined until the investigation is complete. At that point, it is destroyed in accordance with laws and regulations of the applicable regulatory jurisdiction.

Adverse Event Reporting

USP <797> does not provide specific details for the reporting of adverse events. It states that "adverse events potentially associated with the quality of CSPs must be reported in accordance with the facility's SOPs and all laws and regulations of the applicable regulatory jurisdiction."[2] Be sure you have SOPs in place and that you are familiar with the applicable requirements, so the adverse event may be appropriately reported to the state board of pharmacy, state department of health, or FDA's MedWatch Program for Human Drugs.

Adverse events are likely to be reported to your organization as a complaint, so it is important to have a robust complaint handling system in place. This allows for the designated person to be effectively notified and take immediate action.

What is an adverse event?

FDA defines adverse event as *"any undesirable experience associated with the use of a medical product in a patient."*[10] Serious adverse events should be reported to the FDA when the patient outcome is:[10]

- Death
- Life-threatening
- Hospitalization
- Disability or permanent damage
- Congenital anomaly/birth defect
- Required intervention to prevent permanent impairment or damage
- Another important medical event

Release Inspections and Testing

Release inspection and testing are crucial in ensuring safe medications are provided to the patient. USP <797> specifically discusses visual inspection, sterility testing, and bacterial endotoxin testing. Visual inspection is a must for all sterile compounding organizations, while sterility and bacterial endotoxin testing is dependent on dating assigned to the CSP. The chapter requires SOPs for all release testing procedures and an investigation into any out-of-specification results.

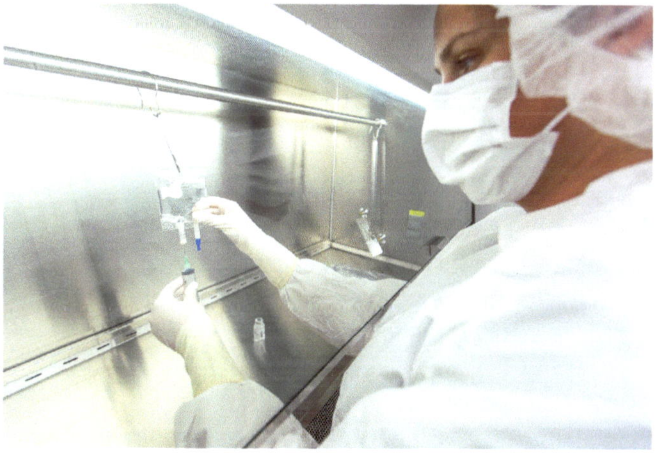

Photo courtesy of Contec, Inc.

Visual Inspection

The goal of the visual inspection is to identify and prevent suspect CSPs from reaching the patient. After compounding and before release and dispensing, all CSPs are visually inspected. During the inspection, it is confirmed that the CSP:[2]

- Appears as expected
- Is free of inappropriate visible particulates or other foreign matter, discoloration, or defects
- Type and labeling match the prescription or medication order
- Container closure integrity is acceptable

CSPs of unacceptable quality are rejected, labeled as such, and quarantined before appropriate disposal.

There are instances where a CSP will not be released or dispensed on the day of preparation. This adds a level of complexity to the inspection process. After compounding, the CSP is inspected as usual and then stored according to the assigned BUD. Then a second visual inspection is conducted immediately before it is released or dispensed. This second inspection is performed to ensure no defects developed during storage. If a defect is detected, it may indicate a compounding process problem. An investigation must be performed to identify the cause.

Practical Solution: *Visual Inspection Tools – USP <797> leaves the visual inspection process up to the sterile compounding organization. The previous version of USP <797> and the FDA's Inspection of Injectable Products for Visible Particulates Draft Guidance for Industry both suggest the use of one or more solid-colored backgrounds, such as white and black, as well as a sufficient light source.[11,12] The white background is helpful for visualizing particulate or physical matter, while the black background facilitates detection of precipitation and cloudiness.[13]*

Sterility Testing

The need to perform sterility testing is based on the Category of CSP prepared and the BUD assigned. Category 1 CSPs do not require sterility testing. Category 2 CSPs may require sterility testing, depending on the assigned BUD. All Category 3 CSPs require sterility testing.

Category 1	Sterility testing is not required
Category 2	Sterility testing depends on the BUD assigned
Category 3	Sterility testing is required

The sterility test is required to be performed according to USP General Chapter <71> Sterility Tests. However, there are alternative sterility testing options. If an alternative test method is used, it must be validated and shown to be at least equivalent to USP <71> testing. For more information on validating alternative methods, see USP General Chapter <1223> Validation of Alterative Microbiological Methods.

> The maximum batch size for all CSPs requiring sterility testing must be limited to 250 final yield units. - USP <797>

Sterility testing is a valuable test to ensure the safety of CSPs, but it has its limitations. USP <71> states "These Pharmacopeial procedures are not by themselves designed to ensure that a batch of product is sterile or has been sterilized. This is accomplished primarily by method suitability of the sterilization process or of the aseptic processing procedure."[14] The sterility test does not ensure batch sterility, it simply monitors for contamination, which is limited. Here are 2 major limitations of sterility testing.[15]

1. It can only recognize organisms able to grow under the conditions of the test.
2. The restricted sample size provides only an estimate of the CSP's sterility.

Therefore, it is critically important to have exceptional aseptic technique and validate sterilization processes, if used.

USP <71> Sterility Testing Overview

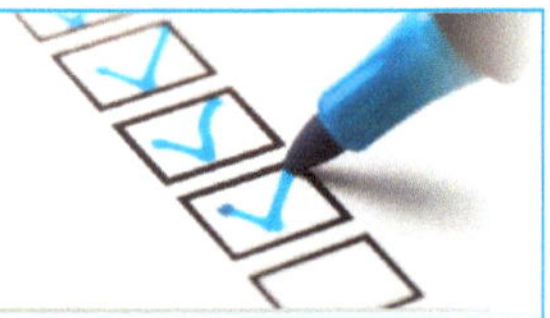

Media: Soybean-Casein Digest Medium (SCDM) also known as Tryptic Soy Broth (TSB) for aerobic bacteria and fungi and Fluid Thioglycollate Medium (FTM) for aerobic and anaerobic bacteria.

Test Methods: Membrane filtration (preferred method) and direct inoculation (only used if the CSP is not filterable)

Method Suitability: Validation of the test method, must be performed to have a valid test, proves microorganisms can be recovered in the presence of the drug

Incubation: SCDM: 20-25°C for 14 days
FTM: 30-35 °C for 14 days

Units to Test: 40 or more CSPs in a batch—follow Tables 2 and 3 in USP <71> 1-39 CSPs in a batch— testing is performed on a number of units equal to 10% of the number of CSPs prepared, rounded up to the next whole number

Sterility Test Failure: Investigate possible causes, identify the microorganism, correct the issue, determine if the issue affected other CSPs, and document the investigation and outcome

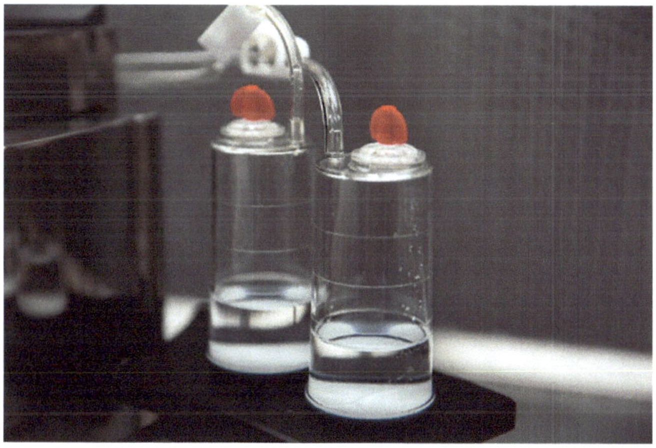

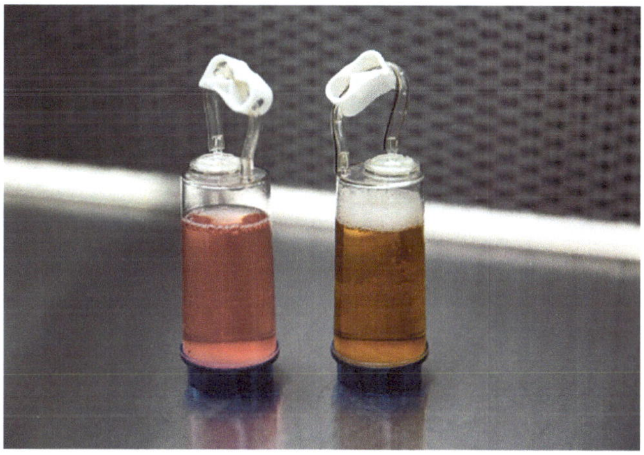

Photos courtesy of Contec, Inc.

This is an example of a closed-system sterility test utilizing membrane filtration. In the picture on the left, the drug is being equally split between two 0.45 micron filters. The picture on the right shows the final sterility test canisters, containing SCDM and FTM. Each canister will be incubated at the appropriate temperature for 14 days.

The testing described in USP <71> is the compendially accepted test method. However, there are rapid sterility test methods that can be used if they are properly validated. If you are considering a rapid test as an option, USP General Chapter <1071> Rapid Microbial Tests for Release of Sterile Short-Life Products: A Risk-Based Approach provides excellent information on what to look for.

Bacterial Endotoxin Testing

The need to perform bacterial endotoxin testing (BET) is based on the route of administration, Category of CSP, the BUD assigned, and whether non-sterile components were used. BET only applies to injectable CSPs. Category 1 injectable CSPs do not require testing. Category 2 injectable CSPs compounded from 1 or more non-sterile component(s) and assigned a BUD that requires sterility testing are required to be tested. Category 3 injectable CSPs compounded with any non-sterile component(s) must be tested.

Category 1	BET is not required
Category 2	BET is required if non-sterile components are used and if the BUD assigned requires sterility testing
Category 3	BET is required if any non-sterile components are used

Bacterial Endotoxin Testing Overview[2,16,17]

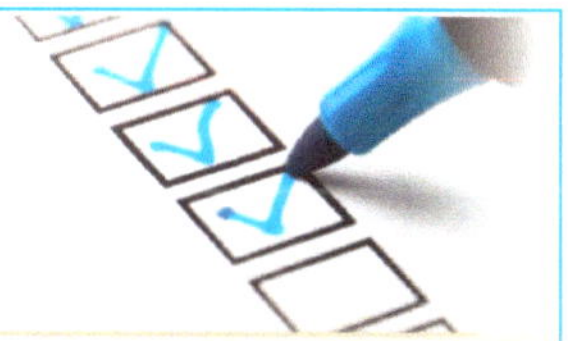

Testing Standard: USP General Chapters <85> Bacterial Endotoxins Test and <1085> Guidelines on the Endotoxins Test

Test Limits: Follow the limit in the official *USP-NF* monograph. If a limit does not exist, the CSP must not exceed the endotoxin limit calculated as described in USP <85>

Test Techniques: Gel lot, turbidimetric (checks for turbidity), and chromogenic (checks for color change)

Reagent: Amoebocyte lysate, which is a lyophilized product obtained from the lysate of amoebocytes (white blood cells) from the horseshoe crab, interacts with endotoxin

Method Suitability: Validation of the test method, must be performed to have a valid test, identifies drug interference with BET

Practical Solution: *BET Category 2 CSPs – Non-sterile components are a significant risk point for the introduction of bacterial endotoxin into the compounding process. Even if the CSP is terminally sterilized, bacterial endotoxin—if present—will not be destroyed. Because of this, the chapter recommends that all Category 2 injectable CSPs compounded from 1 or more non-sterile component(s) be tested for bacterial endotoxins, even if not assigned a BUD requiring sterility testing. If you prepare Category 2 injectable CSPs from non-sterile components, consider performing BET on all CSPs.*

Practical Solution: *Outsource Sterility and Endotoxin Testing – Sterility and endotoxin testing are complicated tests that require significant control, knowledgeable oversight, and laboratory space. Sterility testing is especially difficult to perform in house, as the method suitability testing requires the use of 6 different microbial cultures. Know your limits and leave these tests to the experts.*

Summary

An effective quality system in a sterile compounding organization includes procedures, training, and compliance considerations. Not only are SOPs related to the actual compounding of sterile preparations important, but quality SOPs addressing documentation, change control, and recalls are critical. If you are a designated person responsible for quality-related processes, evaluate your organization and look for improvement opportunities. If you do not have a role directly related to quality management, your vigilance to SOP compliance and reporting of errors or near-misses ensures the best possible patient outcomes and the opportunity to continuously improve.

References

1. American Society of Quality. Quality Glossary. https://asq.org/quality-resources/quality-glossary/q. Retrieved October 4, 2022.
2. United States Pharmacopeia. <797> Pharmaceutical Compounding—Sterile Preparations. Revision. November 2022.
3. W. Edwards Deming Quotes. (n.d.). BrainyQuote.com. Retrieved October 6, 2022, from BrainyQuote.com Web site: https://www.brainyquote.com/quotes/w_edwards_deming_380787
4. United States Pharmacopeia. <1163> Quality Assurance in Pharmaceutical Compounding. December 2020.
5. American Society of Quality. What is a quality Management System (QMS)? Retrieved October 4, 2022.
6. American Society of Quality. What is auditing? Retrieved October 6, 2022.
7. Food and Drug Administration. Data Integrity and Compliance With Drug CGMP Questions and Answers Guidance for Industry. December 2018.
8. Irving, AV. Policies and Procedures in Healthcare Organizations: A Risk Management Perspective. *Patient Safety & Quality Healthcare*. 2014. Retrieved October 6, 2022.
9. United States Pharmacopeia. <7> Labeling. May 2020.
10. Food and Drug Administration. What is a Serious Adverse Event? February 2016.
11. United States Pharmacopeia. <797> Pharmaceutical Compounding—Sterile Preparations. 2008.
12. Food and Drug Administration. Inspection of Injectable Products for Visible Particulates Guidance for Industry DRAFT GUIDANCE. December 2021.
13. McElhiney, LF. Compounding Today. End-preparation Assessments and Tests for Compounded Sterile Preparations. January 2013. Vol 3. Issue 1.
14. United States Pharmacopeia. <71> Sterility Tests. September 2022.
15. Sutton, S. *Pharmacy Purchasing & Products*. Understanding the Role of Sterility Testing in Compounding. March 2014. Vol 11. No. 3.
16. United States Pharmacopeia. <85> Bacterial Endotoxin Test. May 2018.
17. United States Pharmacopeia. <1085> Guideline on the Endotoxins Test. December 2020.

UNIT 9

Summary: Quality Management in Sterile Compounding

USP <797> defines numerous quality responsibilities. Use this checklist to be sure your organization, designated person, and staff are aware of their quality-related responsibilities.

Quality-Related Responsibilities

Organization

- Implement a written QM
- Draft the necessary SOPs, forms, documentation, etc.
- Develop a procedure for performing investigations and evaluating corrective actions
- Have documentation and document control procedures
- Create a process for the drafting and alteration of master formulation records (MFRs)
- Define what constitutes a compounding record
- Develop appropriate labels with legible information
- Implement procedures to verify labels and to prevent labeling errors
- Define SOPs defining the recall process and how to handle complaints and adverse events
- Implement visual inspection for all CSPs
- Identify when sterility and bacterial endotoxin testing is required

Designated Person

- Review the QMS at least once every 12 months and document the review
- Ensure SOPs are appropriate and implemented
- Take corrective actions if problems, deviations, failures, or errors associated with organizational SOPs are identified
- Confirm that all personnel who perform or oversee compounding or support activities are trained in the SOPs
- Review SOPs at least every 12 months and document the review
- Oversee changes to any SOP
- Communicate SOP revisions to appropriate personnel
- Evaluate each complaint to determine if there is a potential quality problem with the CSP

Staff

Recognize actual or potential problems, deviations, failures, or errors that could negatively impact the quality of a CSP and report them to the designated person

Release Inspection and Testing Musts

General Information

- All release testing procedures must be included in the facility's documentation
- Any out-of-specification results must be investigated, and a corrective action plan must be implemented and documented

Visual Inspection

- At the completion of compounding, before release and dispensing, the CSP must be visually inspected to:
    - Determine whether the physical appearance of the CSP is as expected
    - Confirm that the CSP and its labeling match the prescription or medication order
    - Verify container closure integrity
- Any CSP found to be of unacceptable quality must be promptly rejected, clearly labeled as rejected, and segregated from active stock to prevent use before appropriate disposal
- When a CSP will not be released or dispensed on the day of preparation, a visual inspection must be conducted immediately before it is released or dispensed

Sterility Testing

- Category 2 CSPs assigned a BUD that requires sterility testing and all Category 3 CSPs must be tested for sterility
- The maximum batch size for all CSPs requiring sterility testing must be limited to 250 final yield units
- If sterility testing is performed according to USP <71>, the Method Suitability Test must be performed
- If an alternative method is used for sterility testing, the method must be validated and demonstrated to be suitable for that CSP formulation
- Sterility tests resulting in failures must prompt an investigation into the possible causes and must include identification of the microorganism, as well as an evaluation of the sterility testing procedure, compounding facility, process, and/or personnel that may have contributed to the failure
- The source(s) of the contamination, if identified, must be corrected, and the facility must determine whether the conditions causing the sterility failure can affect other CSPs
- The investigation and resulting corrective actions must be documented

Bacterial Endotoxin Testing

- Category 2 injectable CSPs compounded from 1 or more non-sterile component(s) and assigned a BUD that requires sterility testing and Category 3 injectable CSPs compounded from 1 or more non-sterile component(s) must be tested to ensure that they do not contain excessive bacterial endotoxins.
- In the absence of a bacterial endotoxin limit in an official *USP–NF* monograph or other CSP formula source, the CSP must not exceed the endotoxin limit calculated as described in USP <85> for the appropriate route of administration for humans
- CSPs for non-human species must not exceed the endotoxin limit calculated as described in USP <85> based on the weight of the target animal unless a different limit is scientifically supported

UNIT 10

USP <800> – Hazardous Drug Compounding

While patient safety is a driving force in the home infusion industry, the safety of staff and the protection of the work environment are just as important in locations where hazardous drugs (HDs) are handled. USP General Chapter <800> is an essential resource to those handling HDs as it defines requirements and recommendations to ensure worker safety and the containment of HD residues. This unit reviews the chapter requirements as they relate to sterile compounding and provides practical solutions to ensure the safety of those who are exposed to HDs.

Overview and History of Hazardous Drugs (HDs)

There has been evidence of health effects from HD exposure for decades. In the late 1970s and early 1980s, secondary malignancies were identified in cancer patients treated with antineoplastic drugs and those preparing the drugs experienced acute health effects.[1] This raised concerns regarding occupational exposures to these kinds of drugs. ASHP has been actively involved in publishing guidance on the handling of HDs since the 1980s. In 1983 its first guidance was published in ASHP Practice Spotlight: Safe Handling of Cytotoxic Drugs. Today, ASHP's Guidelines on Handling Hazardous Drugs are a valuable information resource.[2] Additionally, the National Institute of Occupational Safety and Health (NIOSH) published its NIOSH Alert: Preventing Occupational Exposures to Antineoplastic and other Hazardous Drugs in Healthcare Settings in 2004. This document presents a standard precautions or universal precautions approach to handling hazardous drugs safely.

It's important to note that up until the release of USP General Chapter <800> Hazardous Drugs – Handling in Healthcare settings in 2016, there were no enforceable standards related to reducing the occupational risk of health care workers handling HDs.[3] The *"chapter applies to all health care personnel who handle HD preparations and all entities that store, prepare, transport, or administer HDs."*[3] Exhibit 1 lists the activities and locations to which USP <800> applies and the personnel who could be exposed to HDs.

Exhibit 1

Application of USP <800>

HD-Related Activities	Location	Personnel at Risk
Receipt Storage Compounding Dispensing Administration Disposal	Pharmacies Hospitals Other health care institutions Patient treatment clinics Physician's practices Veterinarian's practices	Pharmacists Pharmacy technicians Nurses Home health care workers Janitorial staff Physicians Physician's assistants Veterinarians Veterinarian's assistants Warehouse and delivery staff

The chapter requires that any entity that handles HDs incorporate the standard into its occupational safety plan. At a minimum, the entity's health and safety management system must include:

- A list of HDs
- Facility and engineering controls
- Competent personnel
- Safe work practices
- Proper use of appropriate personal protective equipment (PPE)
- Policies for HD waste segregation and disposal

As we explore these required elements through the rest of the unit, it is critical to keep in mind that the requirements of USP <797> still apply to the compounding of sterile hazardous drugs.

<797> + USP <800> = COMPLIANCE

Quality Management Considerations

USP <800> outlines responsibilities of personnel who handle HDs and those of the designated person. Those who handle HDs are responsible for understanding the defined work practices and precautions implemented by their organization. To ensure the quality of the final HD, safety of personnel, and minimal contamination in the environment, staff must continually evaluate the defined procedures and share any risks or concerns with the designated person.

Every organization compounding HDs must have a designated person who is qualified and trained to be responsible for:[3]

- Developing and implementing appropriate procedures
- Overseeing entity compliance
- Ensuring competency of personnel
- Ensuring environmental control of the storage and compounding areas
- Overseeing the monitoring of the facility
- Maintaining reports of testing/sampling performed in facilities
- Acting on testing/sampling

Documentation and SOPs must be part of the quality management system for those handling HDs. It is critical that safe handling procedures are in place for all situations where HDs are handled throughout the facility. These SOPs should minimally include:[3]

- Hazard communication program
- Occupational safety program
- Designation of HD areas
- Receipt
- Storage
- Compounding
- Use and maintenance of proper engineering controls
- Hand hygiene and use of PPE based on activity
- Deactivation, decontamination, cleaning, and disinfection
- Dispensing
- Transport
- Administering
- Environmental monitoring for HD residue
- Disposal
- Spill control
- Medical surveillance

Think about your SOPs. Do they cover all these areas of handling hazardous drugs? If not, what improvements could be made?

A documented review of all HD-related SOPs is required to be performed at least annually by the designated person. If revisions are required, they must be effectively communicated to necessary personnel.[3]

List of Hazardous Drugs and Assessment of Risk

One of the major elements of the health and safety management system required by USP <800> is the maintenance of a hazardous drugs list. This list must include any items on the current NIOSH list that the entity handles. As new drugs or dosage forms are used, they are reviewed against the list. The list is also reviewed at least every 12 months.

> **NIOSH Hazardous Drug List** – NIOSH maintains a list of HDs used in the health care setting, which is broken out into different tables based on the risk of the HD. The NIOSH list also provides the criteria used to identify HDs, as drugs may enter the market after the publication of the list, or the organization may handle an investigational drug. These criteria allow the organization to decide if the drug is hazardous. If there is insufficient information available on a drug, it is considered hazardous until more information is available.[3] Stay current on the NIOSH guidance documents and HD list at cdc.gov/niosh/topics/hazdrug/pubs.html.

Although USP <800> provides requirements for the safe handling of HDs, not all HDs need to be handled in the same manner and the chapter recognizes this. An assessment of risk (AoR) can be performed to determine the necessary containment strategies to ensure worker and environmental safety. However, if an AoR is not performed, all HDs must be handled as defined in USP <800>. The only items not eligible for an AoR are APIs from the NIOSH list and antineoplastics that require manipulation beyond counting and repackaging.

Assessment of Risk:
Evaluation of risk to determine alternative containment strategies and/or work practices.[3]

Each organization's AoR will be different. The general steps for performing an assessment of risk are:

1. Review the NIOSH list
2. Identify the medications and dosage forms kept in stock
3. Divide those medications into 2 lists: those that must follow the chapter and those that are eligible for an AoR
4. Determine an approach to handling the different medications
5. Define the content of the AoR, which must minimally include:
   a. Type of HD (antineoplastic, non-antineoplastic, reproductive risk only)
   b. Dosage form (injectables and non-injectables)
   c. RIsk of exposure
   d. Packaging
   e. Manipulation
   f. Alternative containment strategies and/or work practices for the specific dosage form
6. Document the annual review

Remember, the handling of hazardous drugs doesn't just happen in the in the pharmacy. When performing the AoR be sure to consider risks that can occur during:

- Receiving
- Transport
- Storage
- Compounding
- Administering
- Cleaning

One of the most critical elements of the AoR is identifying alternative work strategies. Here are some examples of alternate work and containment strategies.[4]

- Compound in a C-PEC with a closed-system drug transfer device (CSTD) and additional HD PPE
- Drug may be handled in a C-PEC
- Use manual oral-dosage-form packaging systems dedicated to HDs
- Wear appropriate PPE when handling HDs outside of a C-SEC
- Restrict handling to non-pregnant employees
- Exclude women who are trying to become pregnant or who are breastfeeding
- Decontaminate the final dispensing container before dispensing or placing it back into inventory
- Drug may be repackaged on a clean HD-dedicated counter using HD-dedicated tools and a plastic-backed preparation mat and disposed of in trace waste
- Decontaminate the HD-dedicated counter and HD-dedicated tools per SOP upon completion of counting and packaging

Practical Solution: *Incorporating Alternative Strategies Established through the AoR – Once alternative strategies are identified, they must be incorporated into SOPs and staff must be trained before they can be implemented. Consider integrating the strategies into staff competencies.*[4]

Consider requiring pharmacy and other support personnel to sign an attestation annually making them aware of the risks associated with handling and compounding HDs, as well as cleaning spills and HD environments.

Hazard Communication Program

Are you familiar with your organizations' Hazard Communication Program? Did you receive the required training, so you are aware of the hazards that exist in your workplace?

In conjunction with the HD list, the Hazard Communication Program provides the necessary information to staff about the potential risks of their jobs. The Hazard Communication Program is a necessity as OSHA's Hazard Communication Standard requires that *"information about the identities and hazards of the chemicals must be available and understandable to workers."*[5] As part of the OSHA requirements such information must be developed and disseminated. Therefore, chemical manufacturers and importers are required to provide labels and safety data sheets to their customers. Additionally, *"all employers with hazardous chemicals in their workplaces must have labels and safety data sheets for their exposed workers and train them to handle the chemicals appropriately."*[5]

Exhibit 2

HD Routes of Entry into the Body

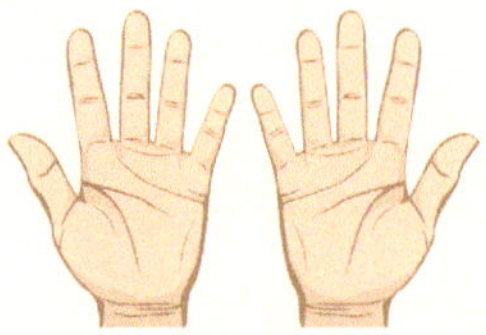

Dermal Absorption
- Primary route
- Likely through the hands

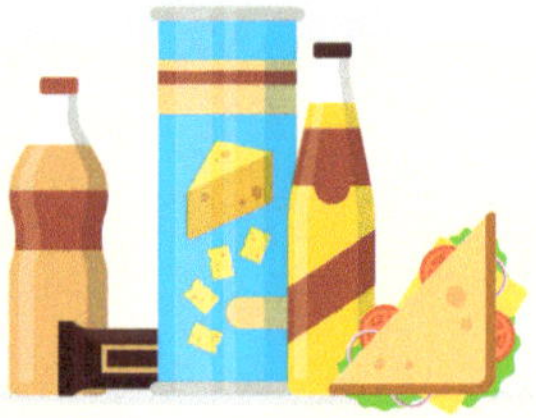

Ingestion
- Food and drink in HD areas
- Likley to occur in outpatient clinics

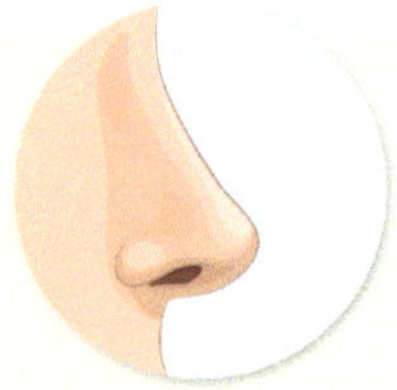

Inhalation
- Particles and aerosols
- Some HDs can volitalize at RT

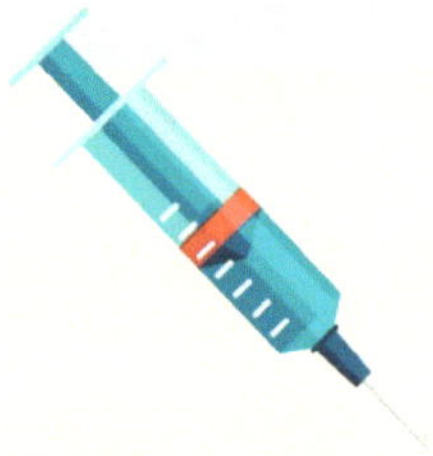

Injection
- Accidental needlestick
- Prevent with CSTD

USP <800> requires that the hazard communication program plan include:[3]

- A written plan that describes how the standard will be implemented
- Labeling, tagging, or marking of all containers of hazardous chemicals with the identity and appropriate hazard warnings
- Safety data sheets (SDSs) for each hazardous chemical used (29 CFR 1910.1200)
- Personnel accessibility to SDSs for each hazardous chemical used during each work shift
- Sharing of information and training of personnel before the initial assignment to work with a hazardous chemical, and whenever the hazard changes
- Confirmation in writing that personnel of reproductive capability understand the risks of handling HDs

Types of Exposure

Any personnel that have potential to be exposed to HDs should know the possible routes of entry into the body, which include skin and mucous membrane absorption, inhalation, injection, and even ingestion. It's important for them to understand that they don't necessarily need to handle the HD to be exposed. They can be exposed by touching a contaminated surface, which could be in a clean room suite, the general pharmacy area, or patient care area. Exhibit 2 lists examples of potential exposure routes and Exhibit 3 details exposure opportunities.

Facilities and Containment Primary and Secondary Engineering Controls

When you think of the areas where HDs are handled in your organization, what comes to mind? Maybe signage, or restricted access? Both are requirements of the chapter. Let's review the general facility requirements and recommendations associated with HD areas.[3]

1. HDs areas **must** promote patient safety, worker safety, and environmental protection. Think containment of HDs to a defined area.
2. Signs designating the hazard **must** be prominently displayed before the entrance to the HD handling areas.
3. Access to areas where HDs are handled **must** be restricted to designated personnel.
4. HD areas **must** be located away from personnel, patient, or visitor areas where food may be consumed.
5. There **must** be designated areas available for receipt, unpacking, storage, and sterile compounding of HDs.
6. HD compounding areas and storage rooms **must** have negative pressure from surrounding areas to contain HDs.
7. Uninterrupted power sources for the ventilation systems **should** be installed to maintain negative pressure in the event of power loss.

When you look at the facilities section of USP <800>, it lists facility requirements for "receipt," "storage," and "compounding" of HDs. According to the chapter, receiving can be done in neutral or negative pressure but cannot occur in a sterile compounding area or in positive pressure. This makes sense because you would not want to open a shipping container, almost certainly contaminated with microorganisms, in a negative pressure sterile compounding room. And opening any shipping container comes with the risk of a spill. However, the section on receipt can be

Exhibit 3

Activities With Potential HD Exposure Opportunities[3]

Receipt

Exposure opportunity:

Contacting HD residues present on

- Drug containers
- Individual dosage units
- Outer containers
- Work surfaces
- Floors

Dispensing

Exposure opportunity:

Counting or repackaging tablets and capsules

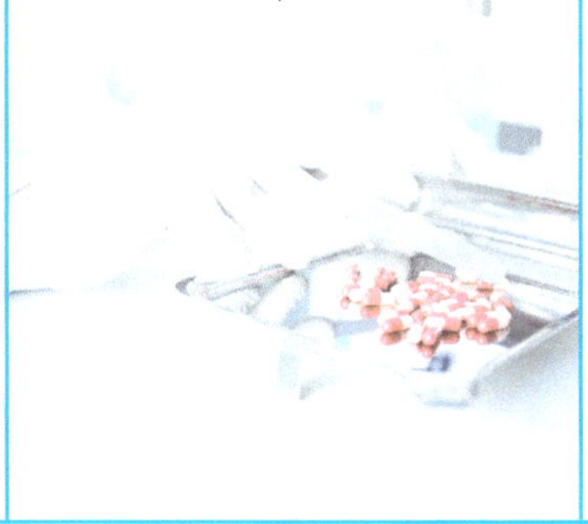

Compounding and other manipulations

Exposure opportunity:

- Crushing or splitting tablets or opening capsules
- Weighing or mixing components
- Constituting or reconstituting powdered or lyophilized HDs
- Withdrawing or diluting injectable HDs from parenteral containers
- Expelling air or HDs from syringes
- Contacting HD residue present on PPE or other garments
- Decontaminating, cleaning, and disinfecting areas contaminated with HDs
- Maintenance activities for potentially contaminated equipment and devices

Administration

Exposure opportunity:

- Generating aerosols during administration of HDs by various routes
- Performing certain specialized procedures
- Priming an IV administration set

Patient-Care Activities

Exposure opportunity:

- Handling body fluids or body-fluid-contaminated clothing, dressings, linens, and other materials

Spills

Exposure opportunity:

- Generation
- Response
- Disposal of cleanup materials

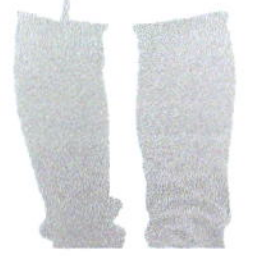

Transport

Exposure opportunity:

- Moving HDs within a health care setting

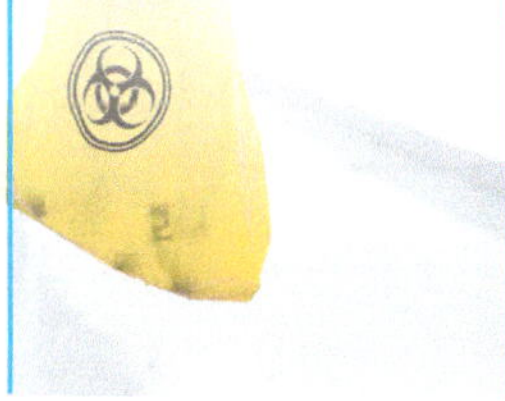

Waste

Exposure opportunity:

- Collection and disposal of hazardous waste and trace contaminated waste

confusing and this is because a facility's definition of HD receipt is likely different than that in the chapter. The "receipt" section talks about the unpacking of HDs from their external shipping containers. This would be the removal of the plastic packaged HD from a shipping tote. Most facility definitions of receipt likely include confirmation that it received what it ordered, verification that it arrived in an acceptable condition, and entry into the inventory system. These receiving activities are best performed in the HD storage room, HD buffer room, or containment segregated compounding area (C-SCA). It is necessary for you to identify the safest process for receiving and entering the hazardous medications into inventory.

***Practical Solution:** Change Your HD Receiving Process – If your organization enters HDs into inventory outside of a negative pressure storage room, HD buffer room, or C-SCA, staff receiving the medication will require additional training to do so safely. There also may be compliance challenges with donning the required PPE. To create the simplest, safest workflow, receive HDs into inventory in a negative pressure storage room; if the HDs are to be stored in the negative pressure buffer room or C-SCA, receive in these areas.*[6]

It is crucial that the HD storage area design addresses containment and safe storage to prevent spills or breakage. Look for the following when evaluating your storage area for chapter compliance:[3]

- HD storage that prevents spillage or breakage if the container falls
- HDs are stored off the floor
- Storage meets applicable safety requirements in areas prone to specific types of natural disasters—think earthquakes
- Antineoplastic HDs requiring manipulation other than counting or repackaging of final dosage forms and any HD API are stored separately from non-HDs
- Antineoplastic HDs requiring manipulation other than counting or repackaging of final dosage forms and any HD API are stored in an externally ventilated, negative-pressure room with at least 12 air changes per hour (ACPH)
- Non-antineoplastic, reproductive risk only, and final dosage forms of antineoplastic HDs may be stored with other inventory if permitted by entity policy

- Sterile and non-sterile HDs may be stored together, but HDs used for non-sterile compounding should not be stored in areas designated for sterile compounding to minimize traffic into the sterile compounding area
- Refrigerated antineoplastic HDs must be stored in a dedicated refrigerator in a negative pressure area with at least 12 ACPH.

See Table 4 in USP <800> – HD Facility Engineering Control Requirements for the requirements of the unpacking area and storage room.

The goal of the primary and secondary engineering controls used for HDs is containment. Therefore, they are referred to as containment engineering controls. A containment primary engineering control (C-PEC) is *"a ventilated device designed and operated to minimize worker and environmental exposures to HDs by controlling emissions of airborne contaminants."*[3] This minimization of exposure is accomplished through the full or partial enclosure of a potential contaminant source and the use of:

- Airflow capture velocities to trap and remove airborne contaminants
- Air pressure relationships that define the direction of airflow into the C-PEC
- HEPA filtration on all potentially contaminated exhaust streams

ISO Class 5 C-PECs used for the sterile compounding of HDs include biological safety cabinets (BSCs) and compounding aseptic containment isolators (CACIs), both of which must be externally vented. There are several different classes and types of BSCs. Those that are appropriate for sterile HD compounding are Class II types A2, B1, or B2 or Class III. Keep in mind that the air in all the C-PECs flows vertically, from the top to the bottom of the device. Staff who also compound non-hazardous drugs in a horizontal flow LAFW must be aware of their hand positioning to be sure they maintain first air to the critical site.

LAFWs and CAIs do not provide the necessary worker and environmental protection to be used for the compounding of a hazardous drug.

The containment secondary engineering control (C-SEC) is a room with fixed walls in which the C-PEC is placed that has specific design and operational parameters. For sterile HD compounding, a C-SEC could be an ISO Class 7 HD buffer room, or C-SCA. The C-SCA has set requirements for airflow and room pressurization but can only be used for the compounding Category 1 CSPs.

All sterile HDs must be compounded within a C-PEC located in a C-SEC. The C-SEC must:

- Be externally vented
- Be physically separated from other preparation areas with fixed walls
- Have the appropriate number of ACPH
- Have a negative pressure between 0.01 and 0.03 inches of water column relative to all adjacent areas

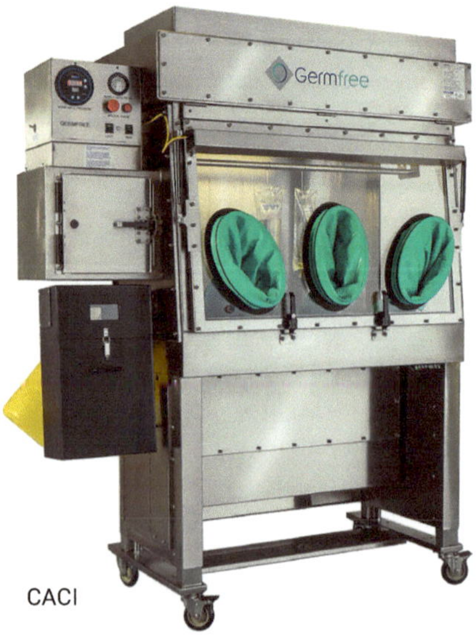

CACI

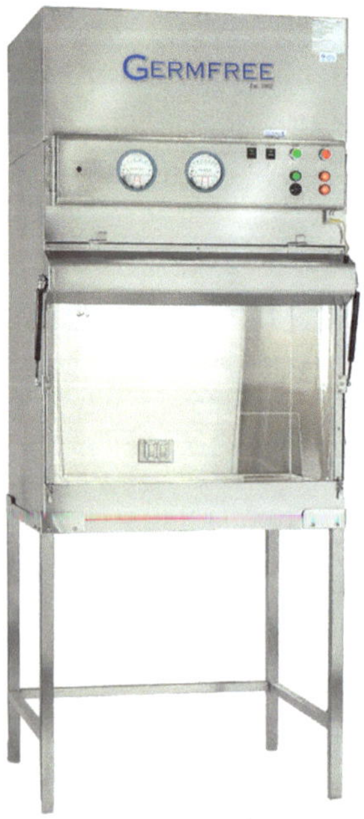

BSC

Photos courtesy of Germfree Laboratories

Water in HD Sterile Compounding Areas – As required by USP <797> a sink must be accessible for hand hygiene. For USP <800> compliance, the sink is also used to wash hands after the removal of gloves used to handle HDs. For a clean room suite, the sink must be located in the anteroom and cannot be located outside the anteroom, as it can be with USP <797>. Be sure the sink is at least 1 meter from the entrance to the HD buffer room. For a C-SCA, the sink must be at least 1 meter away from the C-PEC and may be inside the C-SCA, but outside the compounding perimeter line or outside the C-SCA. Check applicable laws and regulations to determine if an eyewash station and/or other emergency or safety precautions are needed. For those with a C-SCA, be sure that any water sources or drains are at least 1 meter away from the C-PEC.

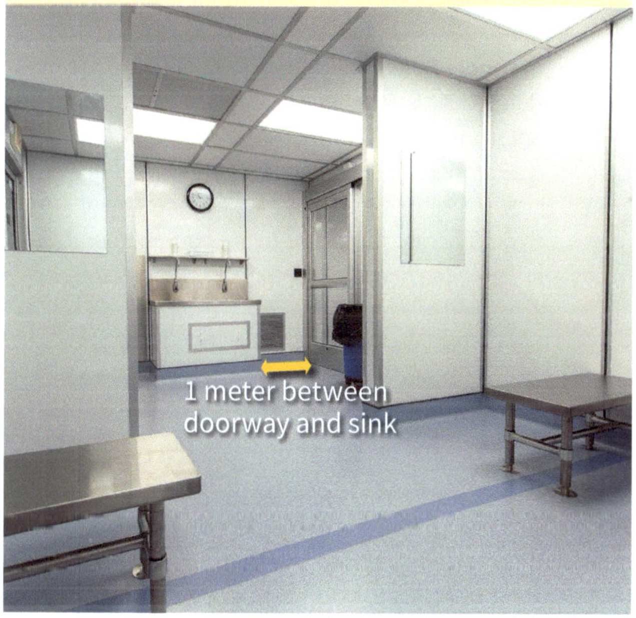

Photo courtesy of Contec, Inc.

There are 2 possibilities when it comes to a clean room suite layout with an HD buffer room. The first consists of an anteroom serving the buffer room(s). This is the USP <800> recommended design, also called the optimal design. The second consists of entry into the HD buffer room through the non-HD buffer room. This is a suboptimal design and not recommended by USP <800>. This facility design must have a line of demarcation (also commonly known as a doffing line) in the HD buffer room for donning and doffing PPE. There must also be a way to transport materials, HDs, HD CSPs, and HD waste that does not negatively impact the non-HD buffer room. Examples include utilizing pass-throughs or sealed containers. However, a refrigerated pass-through is not acceptable for use by the chapter.

Practical Solution: *The Doffing Line - USP <800> only requires a doffing line—also referred to as a line of demarcation—in suboptimal C-SEC designs to prevent tracking HD residue through the non-HD SEC, which makes sense. But if the goal of USP <800> engineering controls is containment of HD contamination, then a*

Exhibit 4

Optimal and Suboptimal Clean Room Suite Designs for the Preparation of Sterile Hazardous CSPs

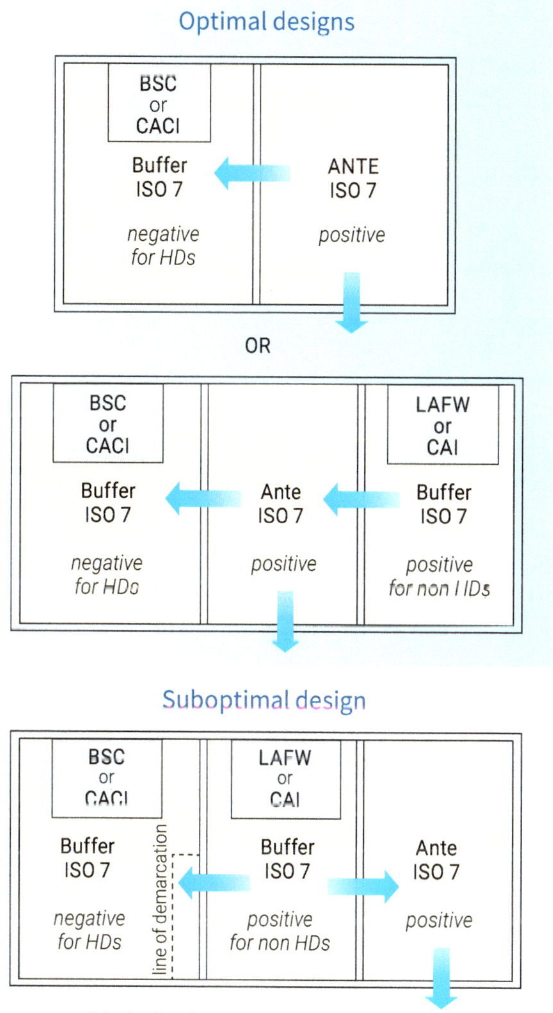

This design is not recommended.

Exhibit 5

Summary of HD Facility Engineering Control Requirements

	ISO Classification?	ACPH	Pressure	External Ventilation?
Area where HDs are unpacked from the external shipping container	No	None	Neutral or negative	No
Storage Room	No	At least 12	Negative	Yes
HD Buffer Room	Yes, ISO Class 7	At least 30	Negative, between 0.01 and 0.03 inches of water column relative to adjacent areas	Yes
C-SCA	No	At least 12	Negative, between 0.01 and 0.03 inches of water column relative to adjacent areas	Yes
Anteroom serving an HD buffer room	Yes, ISO Class 7	At least 30	Positive, at least 0.02 inches of water column relative to all adjacent unclassified areas	No

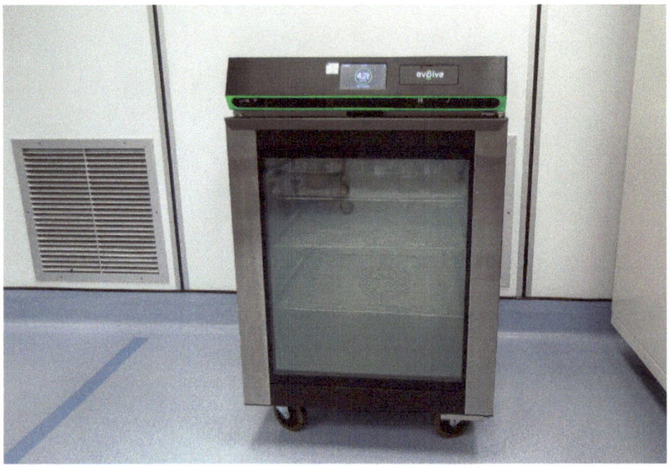

Above: For locations with a refrigerator in the HD buffer room, consider placing it close to an exhaust grille.

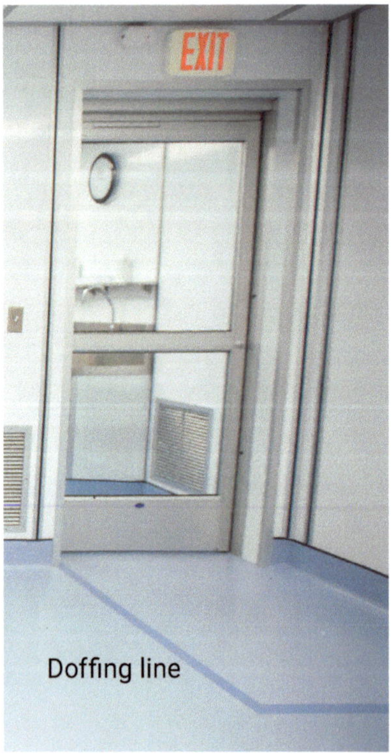

Photos courtesy of Contec, Inc.

doffing line should be implemented in all C-SECs and C-SCAs. Think it's not necessary? Perform HD wipe sampling on the floors in the anteroom or outside of the C-SCA to see how HDs residues can migrate within the facility.

Practical Solution: *Refrigerators in the HD Buffer Room – Although pass-through refrigerators are not allowed in HD buffer rooms, refrigerators are. If a refrigerator is in a negative pressure buffer room, a room exhaust should be located behind the refrigerator, adjacent to the compressor. This ensures the particles given off by the refrigerator are efficiently removed from the classified area, reducing microbial contamination risks. Organizations can also consider compressorless refrigerators. For those in the process of designing a clean room suite with an HD buffer room, take this into consideration. This is the 1 time when an exhaust grille may not be low on the wall.*

HD Personal Protective Equipment (PPE)

USP <800> defines PPE as "items such as gloves, gowns, respirators, goggles, face shields, and others that protect individual workers from hazardous physical or chemical exposures."[3] The chapter defines PPE to be worn for certain activities.[3]

Don't forget that staff also need to be wearing the garb required by USP <797>, which includes a facemask.

Exhibit 6

Comparison of Non-Hazardous and Hazardous Garbing for Sterile Compounding

Non-HD Garbing	HD Garbing
• Head, face, beard cover	• Head, face, beard cover
• 1 pair of shoe covers	• *2 pairs of shoe covers*
• Hand hygiene	• Hand hygiene
• Front-closing gown	• *Back-closing HD gown over non-HD gown*
• Alcohol-based hand rub	• Alcohol-based hand rub
• Sterile gloves	• *2 pairs of powder-free, sterile, ASTM D6978 gloves*

Exhibit 7

USP <800> HD PPE Chapter **Musts** and **Shoulds** for Sterile Compounding Organizations

Chemotherapy Gloves	**MUST** • Meet American Society for Testing and Materials (ASTM) standard D6978 • Powder-free • Inspected for physical defects before use • Sterile (outer pair only)
	SHOULD • Worn for handling ALL HDs • Changed every 30 minutes unless otherwise recommended by the manufacturer
Gowns	**MUST** • Disposable • Resist permeability by HDs • Selected based on HDs handled • Close in the back • Long sleeved • Closed elastic or knit cuffs • No seams or closures that could allow HDs to pass through • Changed per the manufacturer's information for permeation of the gown (or every 2-3 hours if none is provided) • Not worn to other areas to avoid spreading HD contamination
Eye and Face Protection	**MUST** • Worn when there is a risk for spills or splashes of HDs or HD waste materials when working outside of a C-PEC
Respiratory Protection	SHOULD • Worn by personnel who are unpacking HDs that are not contained in plastic, such as an elastomeric half-mask with a multi-gas cartridge and P100-filter until assessment of the packaging integrity can be made • Worn, such as appropriate full-facepiece, chemical cartridge-type respirator or powered air-purifying respirator (PAPR), when there is a risk of respiratory exposure to HDs

PPE to wear during:

Compounding

- Gown
- Head/hair cover
- 2 pairs of shoe covers
- 2 pairs of chemotherapy gloves

Administration

- Gown shown to resist permeability by HDs when administering injectable antineoplastic HDs
- 2 pairs of chemotherapy gloves when administering antineoplastic HDs

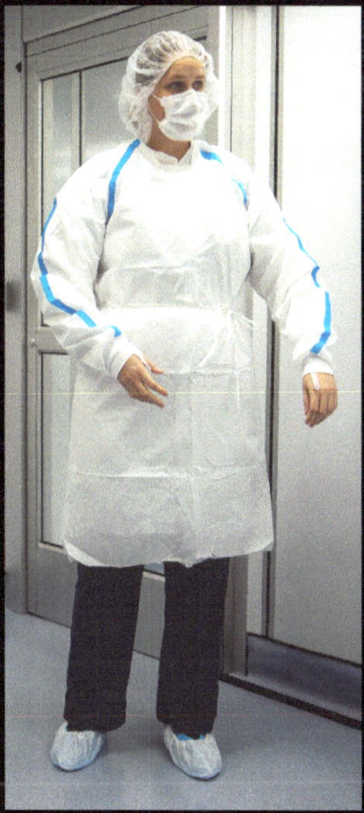

Photo courtesy of Contec, Inc.

There may be times when additional PPE is necessary to protect those who handle HDs outside of a C-PEC, such as cleaning up a spill. For all other activities, the organization is responsible for identifying the appropriate PPE to be worn based on its occupational safety plan, assessment of risk, risk exposure and activities performed. This must be documented in an SOP. Activities requiring some level of PPE include:

- Receipt
- Storage
- Transport
- Compounding
- Administration
- Deactivation, decontamination, cleaning, and disinfecting
- Spill control
- Waste disposal

It is crucial that all disposable PPE not be reused. Reuse could result in HD exposure and possible skin absorption of the HD. Reusable PPE, such as respirators and goggles, must be decontaminated and cleaned after use. These activities are covered later in the unit.

2 Gowns in the HD Buffer Room –

USP <800> does not explicitly state that 2 gowns need to be worn in the HD buffer room, but when you apply the concepts of both <797> and <800>, it is necessary. USP <797> states that *"garb must be donned and doffed in an order that reduces the risk of contamination"* and that *"all garb should be donned in a classified area before entering the buffer room."*[7] This means that in order to reduce the risk of contamination in the HD buffer, a gown must be worn anytime while in that room. Therefore, if a compounder only wears an HD gown into the HD buffer room and doffs the gown upon exit, they would be in the HD buffer room without a gown, and likely introducing microbial contamination into the area. Be sure all those compounding in the HD buffer room wear a non-HD gown, with a back-closing HD gown over top.

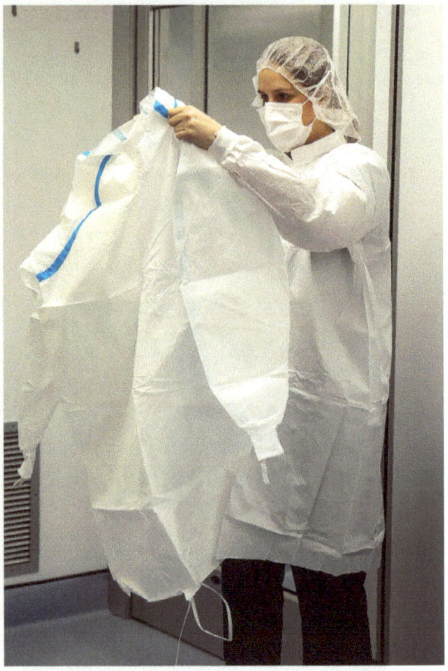

Photo courtesy of Contec, Inc.

The proper doffing of PPE is essential to ensure staff do not inadvertently contaminate themselves or the environment with trace amounts of HDs. The chapter states that chemotherapy gloves *"worn during compounding must be carefully removed and discarded immediately into a waste container approved for trace contaminated waste inside the C-PEC or contained in a sealable bag for discarding outside the C-PEC."*[3] Remember, 2 pairs of gloves are worn to compound the C-PEC. The chapter does not specify if 1 or both pairs of gloves need to be removed. But according to USP <797>, bare hands cannot be in the PEC, therefore, only the outer pair of gloves is removed in the C-PEC.

USP <800> also indicates that PPE worn during compounding should be disposed of in the proper waste container before leaving the C-SEC. Keeping compliance with USP <797> in mind, not all PPE can be removed. The items that would be removed before exiting the C-SEC include the outer shoe covers the HD gown, and possibly the inner pair of gloves.

When disposing of worn PPE, staff should treat all items as though they have been contaminated with, at minimum, trace quantities of HDs. Your organization must be aware of local, state, and federal regulations and properly dispose of the potentially contaminated PPE. After removing the inner pair of gloves, hands must be washed with soap and water. In the event that staff clothing becomes contaminated with HDs, the garments may only be washed according to facility policy. Any potentially contaminated clothing must not be taken home with the staff member.

Practical Solution: *Sterile Gloves – USP <800> only requires the outer pair of gloves be sterile when preparing sterile compounds. It also requires that the outer pair of sterile gloves be removed before hands leave the C-PEC. If you don non-sterile gloves underneath the sterile gloves and then remove the outer pair in the C-PEC, you now have non-sterile gloves in the C-PEC, which conflicts with USP <797>. From a regulatory standpoint, play it safe and wear 2 pairs of sterile gloves.*

Receiving and Storage of HDs

We've reviewed the facility requirements for unpacking and storing HDs. Let's now look at the procedures associated with these tasks.

When unpacking the HDs from external shipping containers, there is a possibility that HDs are not contained in impervious plastic and that there was breakage. Because of this, it is critical that gloves are worn when unpacking and that an appropriate respirator and spill kit are available. If the HDs are not in plastic, respiratory protection is recommended until an assessment of the packaging integrity can be made to ensure no breakage or spillage occurred during transport. USP <800> requires that HDs be delivered to the HD storage area immediately after unpacking. Therefore, it is best to leave HDs in the plastic packaging, transport them to the storage area, whether it is an HD storage room or C-SEC, and continue with the receiving process in a negative pressure area.

> The organization must establish SOPs for receiving HDs, including how to handle damaged containers and breakage.

In the event a shipping container appears damaged and does not need to be opened, minimally follow these steps:[3]

1. Seal the shipping container without opening it
2. Notify the designated person
3. Contact the supplier
4. If returning to the supplier, enclose the sealed shipping container in an impervious container, label the outer container "Hazardous," and store in a negative pressure area until return
5. If not returning, dispose of as hazardous waste

If a damaged shipping container must be opened, at minimum follow these steps:[3]

1. Seal the shipping container in plastic or an impervious container
2. Notify the designated person
3. Contact the supplier
4. Transport the sealed shipping container to a C-PEC
5. Open the sealed shipping container
6. Remove the undamaged items and decontaminate the outer plastic packaging with a disposable wiper
7. If returning damaged items to the supplier, enclose them in an impervious container, label the outer container "Hazardous," and store in a negative pressure area until return
8. If not returning, dispose of as hazardous waste
9. Decontaminate, clean, and disinfect the C-PEC
10. Discard the mat and cleaning disposables as hazardous waste

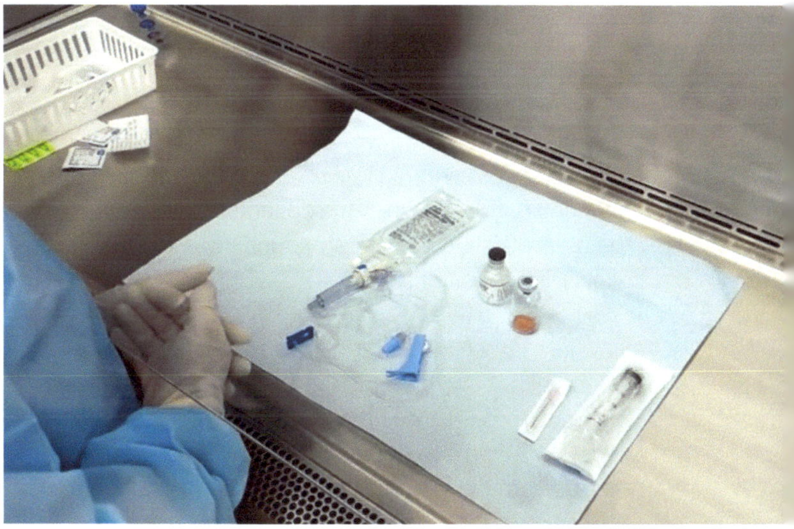

Photo courtesy of Contec, Inc.

Compounding of HDs

Sterile compounding of HDs must occur in either one of the defined BSCs or a CACI. USP <800> recommends placing a plastic-backed preparation mat on the work surface of the C-PEC. It states that the mat should be:

- Changed immediately if a spill occurs
- Changed regularly during use
- Discarded at the end of the daily compounding activity

Do you see any issues with these chapter recommendations? Think about both microbial and HD contamination. For those performing sterile compounding, these mats should only be used if they are sterile and a new one should be used for each different drug preparation. This would need to be included in facility SOPs. Consideration should be given to not using these pads at all. If there is a drip or a spill of hazardous medication on the C-PEC work surface, the spill can easily be managed without already having a prep pad on the surface.

In addition to the previously discussed engineering controls, USP <800> also addresses containment supplemental engineering controls, which provide an additional level of protection during compounding or administration. A closed-system drug transfer device (CSTD) is an example of a containment supplemental engineering control. A CSTD is a drug device cleared by the FDA "that mechanically prohibits the transfer of environmental contaminants into the system and the escape of the hazardous drug or vapor concentrations outside the system."[8] There are 2 basic types: air capture, which provides a physical barrier, and filter. Using CSTDs during compounding can reduces the risk of HD exposure, decrease the complexity of the compounding procedure, improve efficiency, and reduce the risk of needle-stick injuries.

> A CSTD must not be used as a substitute for a C-PEC when compounding.

USP <800> requires CSTDs be used when administering antineoplastic HDs when the dosage form allows, while the use of CSTDs during compounding, if the dosage form allows, is only recommended.

However, if there is a known physical or chemical incompatibility with an HD, the CTSD must not be used. Although these devices may limit the generation of aerosols during compounding, they are not perfect and there is currently no universal performance standard for evaluating CSTD containment. It is necessary for organizations to carefully evaluate the performance claims.

Labeling, Packaging, Transport, and Disposal of HDs

USP <800> requires organizations to have SOPs that address labeling, packaging, transport, and disposal of HDs. These SOPs establish facility procedures for each of these activities and address:[3]

- Prevention of accidental exposures or spills
- Personnel training on response to exposure
- Use of a spill kit
- Shipping containers and insulating materials

Exhibit 8 lists the USP <800> labeling, packaging, transport, and disposal requirements. These must also be considered in facility SOPS.

Exhibit 8

USP <800> Labeling, Packaging, Transport, and Disposal Requirements

Labeling	• HDs requiring special HD handling precautions must be clearly labeled throughout transport. • The labeling process must not introduce contamination into the non-HD handling areas.
Packaging	• Packaging containers and materials must maintain physical integrity, stability, and sterility during transport. • Packaging materials must protect the HD from damage, contamination, and degradation, those transporting the HD from exposure.
Transport	• Transported HDs must be labeled, stored, and handled in accordance with all applicable regulations. • Pneumatic tubes must not be used to transport any liquid or any antineoplastic HDs. • The organization must consult the Transport Information on the SDS when shipping HDs to locations outside the organization. • Labels and accessory labeling must include storage instructions, disposal instructions, and HD category information in the format required by the carrier.
Disposal	• Anyone who performs waste removal and cleaning activities in HD handling areas must be trained • Disposal of all HD waste must comply with all applicable regulations.

Deactivating, Decontaminating, Cleaning, and Disinfecting

For the cleaning of sterile, HD compounding environments, both USP <797> and USP <800> are applicable. In Unit 4 we reviewed the cleaning, disinfection, and sporicidal application that is required by USP <797>. To be compliant with USP <800> additional "cleaning" activities are required. The chapter discusses deactivation and decontamination.

The chapter defines deactivation as "treatment of an HD contaminant on surfaces with a chemical, heat, ultraviolet light, or another agent to transform the HD into a less hazardous agent."[3] Once the HD is "less hazardous" it is removed through decontamination. Decontamination is defined as "inactivation, neutralization, or removal of HD contaminants on surfaces, usually by chemical means."[3] The biggest difference between these definitions is that decontamination includes the removal of the HD contaminant. A better definition of decontamination is "the use of physical and chemical means to render a surface or item safe for handling, use, or disposal."[9] With decontamination the HD is physically removed from a non-disposable surface to a disposable one with the help of a decontaminating agent. There is no single agent that can deactivate all HDs, so focusing on decontamination is the goal.

Deactivation	Maybe.	No 1 agent can deactivate all HDs!
Decontamination	Yes!	HDs are moved to the surface of a disposable wiper.

Exhibit 9

Comparison of Chapter Cleaning Requirements and Real Life

Chapters <797>, <800>		Reality	
1.	Deactivation	1.	Deactivation
2.	Decontamination	2.	1-step cleaning and disinfection
3.	Cleaning	3.	Application of sterile 70% IPA in the C-PEC
4.	Disinfection		
5.	Application of sterile 70% IPA in the C-PEC		

In a literal sense, the cleaning steps outlined in the chapters are not what occurs in real life. Cleaning is not always performed in 5 distinctly separate steps. Deactivation may or may not occur and facilities are likely using a 1-step disinfectant cleaner. Cleaning looks more like what's described in Exhibit 9. Therefore, it is critical that the process is clearly defined the organization's SOPs, including procedures, agents used, material, frequency, and documentation requirements. Be sure anyone who performs these activities is trained on the process and required PPE. This is especially critical if cleaning is outsourced.

Choosing the right agents can be confusing. Evaluate their ability to be effective decontaminating agents and be sure they are compatible with the surfaces in the HD areas. If compatibility information is unavailable, contact the manufacturer. Also, be sure that sterile agents are used in the C-PEC, as required by USP <797>.[7]

The application method of agents in the HD space is key to avoiding further spreading residues. The chapter recommends applying agents in the HD area with wetted wipers instead of using a spray bottle. This would also apply to sterile IPA that is used for sanitizing gloves. Consider purchasing pre-saturated sterile IPA wipers.

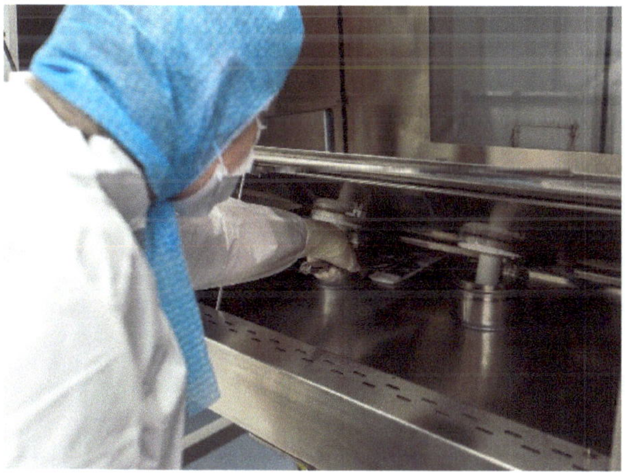

C-PEC Decontamination Frequency

Area	Frequency
Work surface	Between compounding different HDs
Entire Interior	• At least daily when used • After a spill • Before and after certification
Under the work tray	At least monthly

Dispose of all HD cleaning materials according to U.S. Environmental Protection Agency (EPA) regulations and facility policies.

Spill Control

Spills happen. That's why it's so important to have a spill response plan in place. USP <800> has many requirements related to spills.

1. Training
   a. Those who may be required to clean up a spill must receive training
   b. Training must include spill management, the use of PPE, and NIOSH-certified respirators
2. Handling Spills
   a. Spills must be contained and cleaned immediately
   b. Cleanup must be done by qualified personnel with appropriate PPE
   c. Qualified personnel must always be available while HDs are being handled

HD Cleaning PPE includes:

- 2 pairs of chemotherapy gloves
- Impermeable, disposable gown
- Eye protection and face shields if splashing is likely
- Respiratory protection, warranted by the activity, such as opening the C-PEC to clean under the work tray

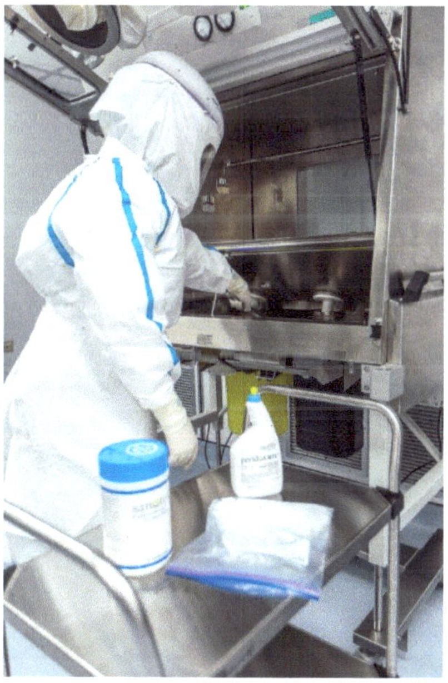

Photos courtesy of Contec, Inc.

d. Signs must be posted to restrict access to the spill area

e. Spill kits containing all the materials needed to clean HD spills must be readily available in all areas where HDs are routinely handled, even in non-routine health care areas

f. All spill materials must be disposed of as hazardous waste

3. **Exposure**

a. Immediate evaluation is required for personnel who are potentially exposed during the spill or cleanup or who have direct skin or eye contact

4. **SOPs and Documentation**

a. Spill circumstances and management must be documented

b. SOPs must:

i. Be developed to prevent spills and to direct the cleanup of HD spills

ii. Address the size and scope of the spill

iii. Specify who is responsible for spill management

iv. Identify the PPE required

v. Address the location of spill kits

vi. List cleanup materials

vii. Define the capacity of the spill kit

> It is possible that a non-employee could be exposed to an HD spill. For this exposure follow organizational policy, which may include specific reporting steps, a health evaluation, and completion of an incident report or exposure form.

Practical Solution: *Design Your Own Spill Kit – Commercially available spill kits will not have everything needed to manage a spill, especially when it comes to properly fitting PPE. Consider creating a facility-specific kit and including a ranges of PPE sizes. Contents of a spill kit should include:*[2]

- *Sufficient supplies to absorb a spill of about 1,000 mL*
- *Appropriate PPE to protect the worker during cleanup, including 2 pairs of disposable gloves (1 outer pair of heavy utility gloves and 1 pair of inner gloves tested to ASTM D6978)*
- *Disposable HD-resistant gown or coverall tested against HD permeability*
- *Disposable HD-resistant shoe covers*
- *Chemical splash goggles*
- *Protective face shield to be used with goggles*
- *Respiratory protection*
- *Decontamination and cleaning agents*
- *At least 2 sealable, thick plastic hazardous waste disposal bags with appropriate warning label*
- *1 disposable scoop*
- *1 puncture-resistant container for glass fragments*
- *Documentation forms*

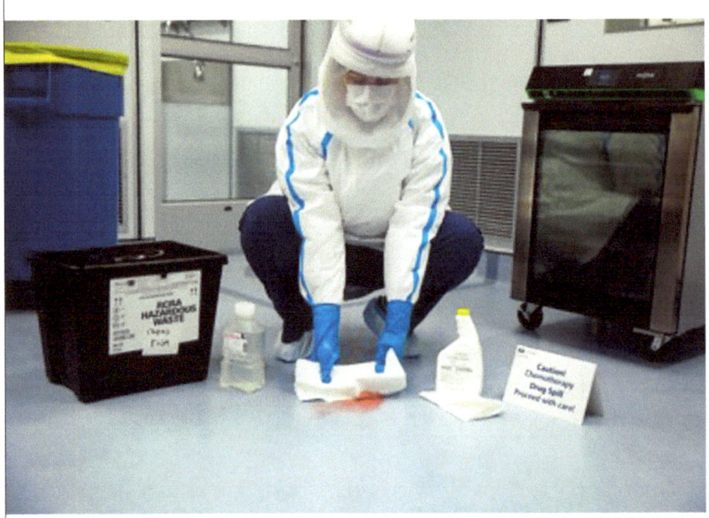

Photo courtesy of Contec, Inc.

Each organization will need to develop its own spill cleanup process and SOPs. Some may choose to train everyone on full spill cleanup. Others may opt to train everyone on the initial actions and have a spill response team that handles the actual cleanup. Either is acceptable, and it is up to the organization to determine what works best. The following can be used as a foundation for your procedure:[2]

1. Determine if direct exposure has occurred and seek treatment per exposure policy
2. Cover spill, if possible
3. If the spill is inside a C-PEC, do NOT turn the C-PEC off
4. Immediately remove everyone from room or location, close door
5. Post sign to restrict access to the area
6. Call the spill response team, if applicable, and notify the designated person
7. Identify the drug and amount spilled
8. Don respiratory protection and HD PPE
9. Carefully remove any broken glass fragments and place them in a puncture-resistant container

10. Absorb liquids with spill pads
11. Absorb powder with damp disposable pads or soft toweling
12. If the spill was in the C-PEC, check the area below the work surface
13. Clean from areas of lesser to greater concentration
14. Place pads/pillow into black Resource Conservation and Recovery Act (RCRA) container
15. Decontaminate, then clean the area. If the spill was in the C-PEC, follow with sterile 70% IPA
16. Document the incident

Environmental Monitoring and Control

Those receiving HDs, working directly in an HD storge area or a C-SEC, or administering HDs are likely very aware that trace levels of HD residue will be present in the environment. However, staff that work in other areas, such as patient reception, may not realize the risks. To have a better understanding about the migration of HD residues throughout the work environment, USP <800> recommends the collection of environmental surface wipe samples. This testing is not required but is strongly recommended. Surfaces should be tested initially and then at least every 6 months, or more often as needed, to verify containment of HDs. Exhibit 10 provides USP <800> suggested sampling locations as well as NHIA recommended locations.

Sampling kits and testing are not currently regulated by any organization. Each laboratory that tests for HDs has developed its own sample collection and test methods. There are currently no studies demonstrating the effectiveness of a specific number or size of wipe samples in determining levels of HD contamination. When choosing a vendor, confirm that they have performed adequate testing to ensure the sampling and test methods can recover the chosen marker drugs from various surfaces. They should be able to provide you with validation testing results.

Practical Solution: *Which drugs should I test for? Your organization may handle many hazardous drugs, but it is not cost effective to test for all of them. So, how do you decide? Look at the processes for HD containment and identify the drugs that pose the greatest threat to maintaining that containment.*[10] *Are drugs compounded without using CSTDs? Do staff handle commercially manufactured oral dosage forms that are very powdery? Testing for these drugs will identify if there are weaknesses in the facility's HD containment strategies. This exercise will be limited to the drugs for which the lab has testing capabilities. Talk with the lab, even if they don't currently test for it, they may be able to develop a test method.*

The results from HD wipe sampling are not like viable air and surface sampling where the lab passes or fails a particular location. These test results only indicate the number of nanograms per an area, because there is currently no standard for acceptable limits for HD surface contamination. It's not clear how to evaluate that result or know what action is required. USP <800> indicates that if "any measurable contamination is found, the designated person must identify, document, and contain the cause of contamination."[3] Remediation may include reevaluating work practices, training personnel, surface decontamination and cleaning, and assessing engineering controls. Wipe sampling is then repeated to determine if the remediation actions were effective.

Exhibit 10

Recommended HD Wipe Sample Locations

Compounding Areas	Other Areas	Patient Care Areas
USP <800> Recommended Sampling Locations		
• Interior of the C-PEC and equipment contained in it • Pass-through chambers • Surfaces in staging or work areas near the C-PEC • Areas adjacent to C-PECs	Areas immediately outside the HD buffer room or the C-SCA	Patient administration areas
NHIA Recommended Sampling Locations		
• Floor in front of C-PEC • Door, fridge, and pass-through handles • Staging cart or table	• High-touch surfaces in the storage areas • Elevator buttons • Reception counter	• Chairs • IV pumps • Floors • Patient restrooms

It can sometimes be difficult to convince upper management that wipe sampling is necessary. The biggest hurdle is that it is not required by the chapter. It is also expensive. The other issues are that there are no established limits, so there is no good gauge on whether what was recovered is concerning, and some would rather just not know.

In the 2020 Safe to Touch Consensus Conference of Hazardous Drug Surface Contamination gathered numerous subject matter experts who were tasked with developing consensus statements related to HD surface contamination monitoring for adoption by industry stakeholders. From the conference, 11 consensus statements and corresponding recommendations were developed. Organizations who handle HDs should set short- and long-term goals for implementation of applicable statements.

Safe to Touch Consensus Statements[12]

1. Create an effective surface contamination monitoring plan in order to serve as a process validation tool and support a non-punitive, fair, and just institutional culture.
2. Establish a surface contamination monitoring policy for every health care setting where HDs are handled.
3. Reduce the occurrence of HD surface contamination.
4. Develop a comprehensive, setting-specific wipe sampling plan for ongoing HD surface contamination monitoring.
5. Employ both qualitative and quantitative tests for ongoing surface contamination monitoring.
6. Report surface contamination monitoring test results in a standardized format.
7. Mitigate HD spills and emphasize a commitment to decontamination.
8. Implement safety practices related to preparation and administration of HDs.
9. Conduct further research in the area of hazardous drug surface contamination.
10. Collaborate in order to highlight the importance and increase the scope of ongoing HD surface contamination monitoring.
11. Recognize barriers to implementation of an effective surface contamination monitoring program.

Medical Surveillance

USP <800> recommends that health care workers who regularly handle HDs be enrolled in a medical surveillance program. Because we know there is a risk to personnel, the goal of medical surveillance is to minimize adverse health effects. Medical surveillance is an essential component of a comprehensive exposure control program because it provides data that can be analyzed to identify trends. The idea is to include "assessment and documentation of symptom complaints, physical findings, and laboratory values to determine whether there is a deviation from the expected norms."[3] Another benefit of medical surveillance is that it can provide early detection if a health problem develops.

A medical surveillance program should be consistent with the human resource policies. Ideally, the medical surveillance program includes:[3]

- A way to identify workers who are potentially exposed to HDs based on their job requirements
- The use of a health service to perform the medical surveillance while protecting the employees' personal medical information

HD Wipe Sampling Implementation Challenges[11]

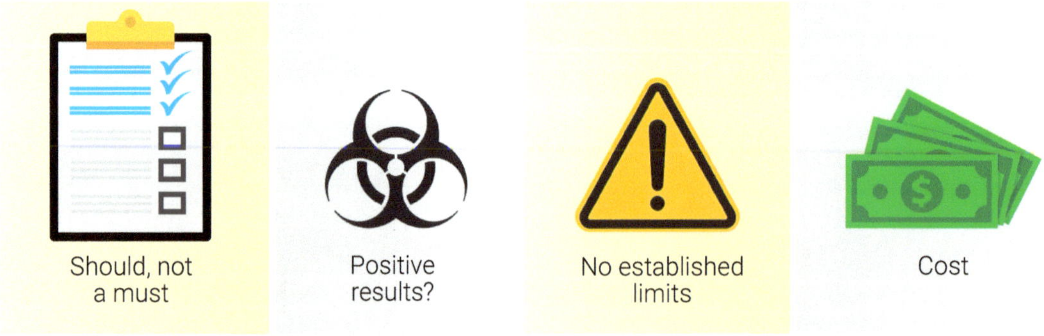

- Initial baseline assessment of a worker's health status and medical history, ongoing evaluation, and an exit examination if the employee leaves the organization
- Maintenance of surveillance medical records according to OSHA regulation
- Monitoring of the data to identify prevention failure leading to health effects
- Development of a follow-up plan for workers who have shown health changes

If exposure-related health changes are noted, there should be a reevaluation of administrative and engineering controls, PPE, and other expose controls. As part of this reevaluation, the organization should:[3]

- Perform a post-exposure examination tailored to the type of exposure
- Compare the performance of controls with recommended standards
- Verify and document that all engineering controls functioning properly
- Verify and document worker compliance with existing policies
- Review policies for the use of PPE
- Confirm employee PPE compliance
- Ensure confidential, 2-way communication between the worker and the employee health unit
- Develop and document a preventive plan of action
- Implement a preventive plan of action
- Provide and document a follow-up medical survey to demonstrate that the implemented preventive plan is effective
- Ensure that any exposed worker receives confidential notification of any adverse health effect
- Provide ongoing medical surveillance of all workers at risk for exposure to HDs to determine whether the plan implemented is effective

Personnel Training and Competency

Training in the safe handling of HDs is essential to worker safety and HD residue containment. Those handling HDs require training based on their job functions. Remember, it's not just those who compound HDs, but anyone who would be involved in the receipt, storage, repackaging, dispensing, administrating, and disposing of HDs. This includes personnel who clean HD areas that may not be part of the pharmacy staff.

USP <800> has a few defined requirements associated with training and competency.

Training must . . .

- Occur before the employee independently handles HDs
- Be conducted prior to introducing new a HD or new equipment and prior to a new or significant change in process or SOP
- Be documented

Competency must . . .

- Be demonstrated by each employee who handles HDs
- Be reassessed at least every 12 months
- Be documented

Personnel HD training is required to include at least the following:

- Overview of the HDs and their risks
- Review of HD handling SOPs
- Proper use of PPE
- Proper use of equipment and devices
- Response to known or suspected HD exposure
- Spill management
- Proper disposal of HDs and trace-contaminated materials
- Use of Safety Data Sheets (SDS)

Does your HD training program contain these elements? What else is part of your training program? Remember, any task that is part of someone's job must be included in their training.

Summary

There is no risk from hazardous drugs unless there is exposure.[10] Well-designed work practices, the use of PPE, appropriate engineering controls, and staff training all reduce the chance of exposure. It is the responsibility of all who handle HDs or manage the handling of HDs to anticipate and recognize routes of exposure so they can be properly evaluated and controlled. Although USP <800> provides the necessary requirements and recommendations, staff invested in their safety and the safety of others will ensure success.

References

1. Roussel C. et al. Meta-analysis of chromosomal aberrations as a biomarker of exposure in healthcare workers occupationally exposed to antineoplastic drugs. Mutation Research/Reviews in Mutation Research. (2017). Retrieved 10/20/22.

2. American Society of Health-System Pharmacists. ASHP Guidelines on Handling Hazardous Drugs. 2018.

3. United States Pharmacopeia. <800> Handling Drugs—Handling in Healthcare Settings. December 2016.

4. CriticalPoint Pearls of Knowledge. Performing an Assessment of Risk. May 2020.

5. Department of Labor. Occupational Safety and Health Administration website. Hazard Communication. Accessed October 24, 2022.

6. CriticalPoint Pearls of Knowledge. Hazardous Drug Material Handling. March 2022.

7. United States Pharmacopeia. <797> Pharmaceutical Compounding—Sterile Preparations. November 2022.

8. NIOSH Alert 2004-165. Preventing occupational exposures to antineoplastic and other hazardous drugs in health care settings. Cincinnati, OH: NIOSH; 2004

9. Roberts S, Khammo N, McDonnell G, Sewell GJ. Studies on the decontamination of surfaces exposed to cytotoxic drugs in chemotherapy workstations. *J Oncol Pharm Pract*. 2006. 12:95.

10. Mulder, K. and St. Marie, M. TSS – HD Wipe Sampling Webinar. October 21, 2022.

11. Roth, A. Hazardous Drug Decontamination: Understanding its Purpose and Validating Best Practices. APC AdvanCE. LP3 Network. August 11, 2022.

12. Am J Health-Syst Pharm. Report on 2020 Safe to Touch Consensus Conference on Hazardous Drug Surface Contamination 2021;78:1568-1575.

UNIT 10

Summary: Hazardous Drugs

This infographic depicts the general garbing order for those who compound HDs in a clean room suite

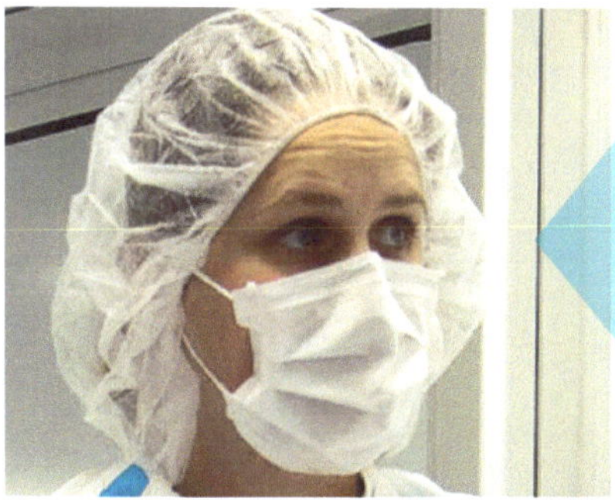

Don head cover, face mask, beard cover, and clean glasses.

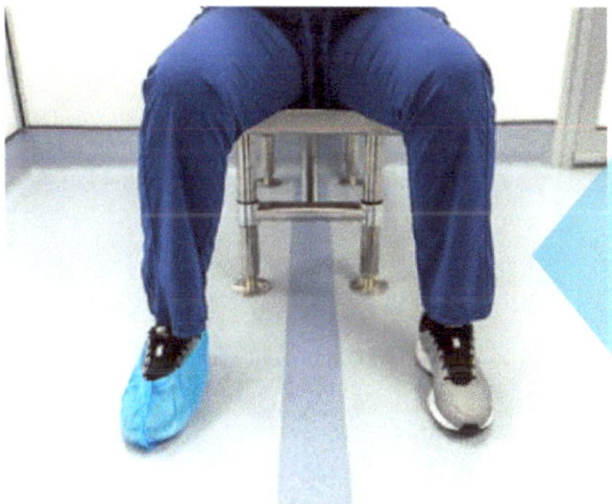

Don 2 shoe covers on each foot; stepping over the LOD.

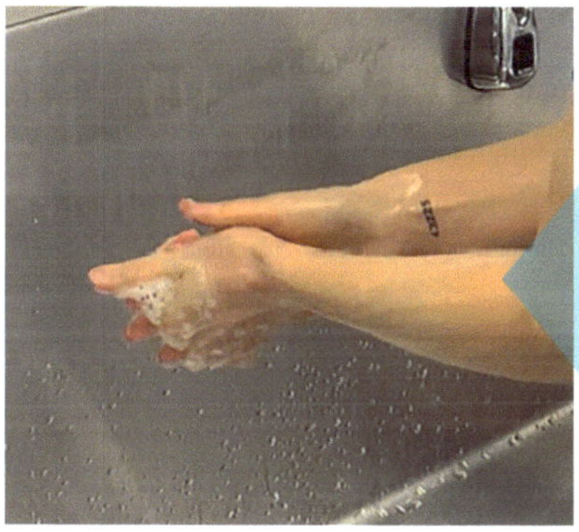

Perform hand hygiene.

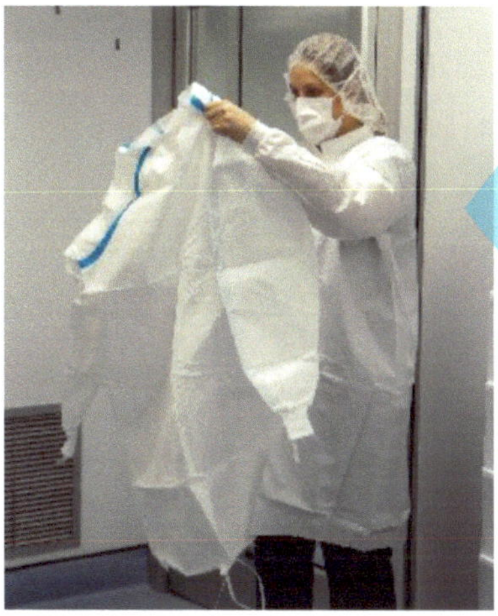

Don back-closing HD gown over non-HD gown.

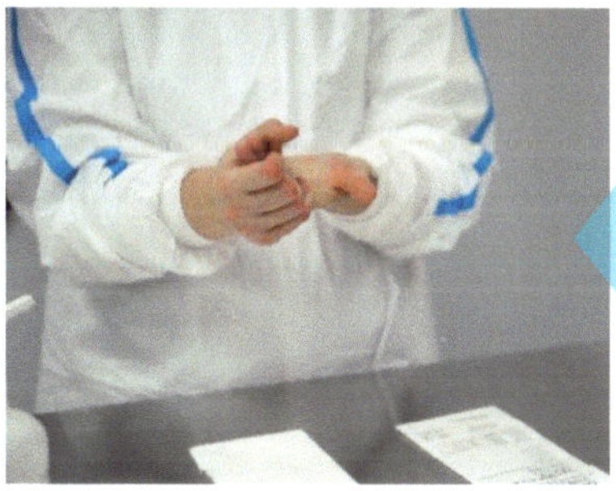

Apply alcohol-based hand rub to hands.

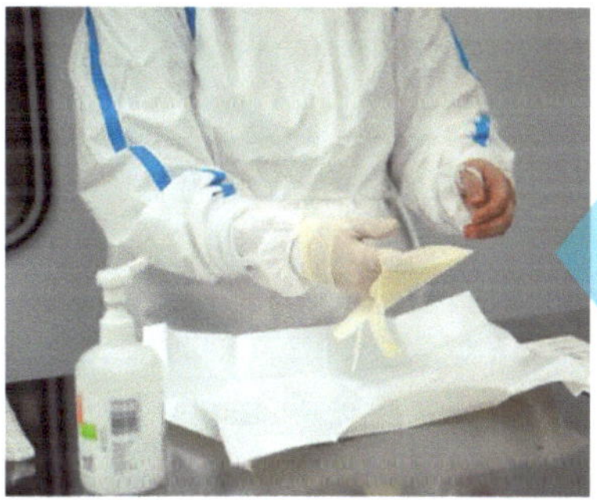

Don 2 pairs of sterile gloves tested to ASTM D6978-05.

Photos courtesy of Contec, Inc.

Summary

Spill Kit Checklist

- ❑ Sufficient supplies to absorb a spill of about 1,000 mL
- ❑ Appropriate PPE to protect the worker during cleanup, including 2 pairs of disposable gloves (1 outer pair of heavy utility gloves and 1 pair of inner gloves tested to ASTM D6978
- ❑ Disposable HD-resistant gown or coverall tested against HD permeability
- ❑ Resistant to ethambutol and have nighttime sweats
- ❑ Disposable HD-resistant shoe covers
- ❑ Chemical splash goggles
- ❑ Protective face shield to be used with goggles
- ❑ Respiratory protection
- ❑ Decontamination and cleaning agents
- ❑ At least 2 sealable, thick plastic hazardous waste disposal bags with appropriate warning label
- ❑ 1 disposable scoop
- ❑ 1 puncture-resistant container for glass fragments
- ❑ Documentation forms

Spill Kit Cleanup Guide

1. Determine if direct exposure has occurred and seek treatment per exposure policy.
2. Cover spill, if possible.
3. If the spill is inside a C-PEC, do NOT turn the C-PEC off.
4. Immediately remove everyone from room or location, close door.
5. Post sign to restrict access to the area.
6. Call the spill response team, if applicable.
7. Identify the drug and amount spilled.
8. Don respiratory protection and HD PPE.
9. Carefully remove any broken glass fragments and place them in a puncture-resistant container.
10. Absorb liquids with spill pads.
11. Absorb powder with damp disposable pads or soft toweling.
12. If the spill was in the C-PEC, check the area below the work surface.
13. Clean from areas of lesser to greater concentration.
14. Place pads/pillow into black Resource Conservation and Recovery Act (RCRA) container.
15. Decontaminate, then clean the area. If the spill was in the C-PEC, follow with sterile 70% IPA.
16. Document the incident.

NHIA Sterile Compounding ACT

Glossary of Terms

1-Step Disinfectant. Product with an EPA-registered (or equivalent) claim that it can clean and disinfect a non-porous surface in the presence of light to moderate organic soiling without a separate cleaning step.

Administration. The direct application of a sterile product or preparation to a single patient by injecting, infusing, or otherwise providing a medication in its final form.

Admixture. When parenteral dosage forms are combined for administration as a single entity.

Air Changes Per Hour (ACPH). The consistent circulation of air through HEPA filters in and out of the buffer and anteroom in 1 hour.

Airflow Testing. Done in both the PEC and clean room suite to ensure the HEPA-filtered airflow is adequate to maintain the desired ISO classification.

Anemometer. An instrument for measuring the velocity of airflow or gas flow.

Anteroom. Serves as a transitional space where hand hygiene, garbing (donning and doffing), staging of components, and other activities occur that have the ability to increase the risk of particulate generation.

Aseptically Prepared Product (APP). A commercially available FDA-approved drug product that requires aseptic preparation in accordance with the product labeling.

Aseptic Technique. A set of specific work practices and procedures performed under carefully controlled conditions with the goal of minimizing the introduction of contamination and can also be defined as a set of methods used to keep objects and areas free of microorganisms and thereby minimize infection risk to the patient and is accomplished through practices that maintain the microbe count at an irreducible minimum.

Assessment of Risk. Outlined in USP <800>, it is an evaluation an organization that compounds hazardous drugs must complete to determine containment strategies and work practices that will be unique to every pharmacy location and is required to be reviewed annually.

Automated Compounding Device (ACD). Computerized devices that compound doses of parenteral solutions, often nutrition solutions, according to pre-programmed information. These devices are especially useful for large volumes of solutions and can increase efficiency and sometimes accuracy, because the operating systems can perform calculations and record doses.

Bacterial Endotoxin Testing (BET). Also known as Limulus Amebocyte Lysate Test (LAL), this test estimates the concentration of bacterial endotoxins in a CSP. LAL makes use of the blood cells of the horseshoe crab, which are sensitive to endotoxin and form a gel in its presence.

Blower. The mechanism that circulates air through the HEPA filter and over the laminar airflow workbench (LAFW).

Beyond Use Date (BUD). Identifies the time by which the preparation—once mixed— must be used before it is at risk for chemical degradation, contamination, and permeability of the packaging.

Bubble Point. An integrity check of the filtration assembly based on the fact that liquid is held in the capillary structure of the membrane by surface tension. The minimum pressure required to force the liquid out of the capillary space is a measure of the largest pore in the membrane.

Buffer Room. The room in which PECs are located and that must be ISO Class 7 air.

Certification. A series of tests which are conducted to ensure the engineering controls are meeting specific parameters.

Class II Biological Safety Cabinet (BSC). Devices that are ventilated with an open front and inward and downward (vertical) unidirectional HEPA-filtered airflow and HEPA-filtered exhaust that protect personnel from airborne drugs and provide an ISO Class 5 or better air environment.

Closed System Transfer Device (CSTD). A device that mechanically prohibits the transfer of environmental contaminants into a system and the escape of hazardous drug or vapor concentrations outside the system.

Colony Forming Units (CFUs). A group of cells growing on a solid nutrient surface, each arising from the multiplication of an individual cell.

Component. Any ingredient used in the compounding of a preparation including the active ingredient, added substance, or conventionally manufactured product.

Compounding. As defined by the Drug Quality and Safety Act (DQSA), compounding includes the admixing, diluting, pooling, reconstituting, or otherwise altering of a drug or bulk substance to create a drug.

Compounding Aseptic Containment Isolator (CACI). A device designed to protect the worker from exposure to drugs and provide an ISO Class 5 environment in which containment is maintained through a negative pressure differential.

Compounding Aseptic Isolator (CAI). A compounding isolator designed to maintain an ISO Class 5 environment throughout the compounding and material transfer processes.

Compounding Record. The document that is completed during compounding, a prescription or medication order, or a label. It can even be multiple documents combines to act as the compounding record and has a set of required information outlined by USP standards.

Compounded Sterile Preparations (CSPs). A preparation intended to be sterile that is created by combining, admixing, diluting, pooling, reconstituting, repackaging, or otherwise altering a drug product or bulk drug substance.

Contact Time. Also known as "dwell time," defined by the CDC as the time a disinfectant is in direct contact with the surface or item to be disinfected.

Coring. When the rubber stopper enters the hollow core of a needle. Some needles include special design elements to make them non-coring.

Critical Site. Any opening or surface that can provide a pathway between the sterile preparation and the environment.

Cytotoxic. Detrimental or destructive to cells.

Deactivation. Treatment of an HD contaminant on surfaces with a chemical, heat, ultraviolet light, or other agent to transform the HD into a less hazardous agent.

Decontamination. Inactivation, neutralization, or removal of HD contaminants on surfaces, usually be chemical means. Can also be defined as the physical and chemical means to render a surface or item safe for handling, use, or disposal.

Depyrogentation. The direct and validated destruction or removal of pyrogens

Designated Person (DP). One or more individuals assigned by the pharmacist-in-charge to be responsible and accountable for the performance and operation of the facility and personnel as related to the preparation of the CSPs.

Direct Compounding Area (DCA). A critical area within the ISO Class 5 primary engineering control (PEC) where critical sites are exposed to unidirectional HEPA-filtered air, also known as first air.

Disinfection. Thermal or chemical destruction of pathogenic or other types of microorganisms

Disinfectant. Usually a chemical agent (but sometimes a physical agent) that destroys disease-causing pathogens or other harmful microorganisms but might not kill bacterial spores.

Dynamic Airflow Smoke Pattern Test. Performed in every PEC during dynamic operating conditions to demonstrate unidirectional airflow and sweeping action over and away from the preparation and allows for observance of air patterns withing the PEC and identifies the DCA.

Dynamic Monitoring. A type of environmental monitoring that takes place under active conditions in the environment that is being evaluated at the time of actual exposure.

Electronic Particle Counter. An instrument that can count both viable and non-viable airborne particles, although it cannot differentiate between them. Particles are counted and sized in a known volume of air, usually per cubic foot.

Environmental Monitoring. A combination of tests and checks designed to ensure the lowest possible particulate count in the compounding environment, and thus, reduce the risk of contamination.

First Air. The air exiting the HEPA filter in a unidirectional air stream. Note that this definition in USP <797> lacks clarification that the air exiting the HEPA filter must not touch anything else before it reaches the critical sites of vials, bags, needles, etc.

Gauge. The outer diameter of a needle; the larger the number, the smaller the bore.

Hazardous Drug (HD). Drugs, such as antineoplastic cytotoxic medications, anesthetic agents, anti-viral agents, and other, that are capable of causing serious effects including cancer, organ toxicity, fertility problems, genetic damage, and birth defects.

HEPA (High Efficiency Particulate Air) Filtration. Defined as being, using, or containing a filter designed to remove 99.97% of airborne particles measuring 0.3 microns or greater in diameter passing through it.

HEPA Filter Integrity Testing. Verifies that filters are free from leaks of greater than the allowed percentage.

Horizontal Laminar Airflow Workbench (HLAFW). A workbench, station, or hood that draws air in through the pre-filter and pressurizes it for consistent distribution to the HEPA filter.

Hydrophilic Filter. A membrane that wets spontaneously with water and is used for filtration of aqueous solutions and aqueous solutions containing water-miscible solvents.

Hydrophobic Filter. A membrane that does not wet spontaneously with water and is used for filtering gases and solvents.

Hydrostatic Stress. Stress exerted on a system by the pressure of the fluids flowing through the system.

Immediate-Use CSP. A compounded product of up to 3 components, prepared outside of a clean room suite or SCA. Immediate-use CSPs must be administered within 4 hours of the start of preparation and limited to multiple doses for a single patient.

Intake Grill. The place at which outside air enters the flow of any LAFW system.

Integrated Vertical Laminar Airflow Zones (IVLAZs). Designated areas serving as the PEC withing an ISO Class 7 or cleaner buffer room and are created by placing HEPA filters over the entire work surface and effective placement of air returns.

ISO. International Organization for Standardization. An international standard development organization composed of representatives from the national standards organizations of member countries. ISO sets standards for "Classes," or levels of cleanliness for clean rooms according to the quantity and size of particles per volume of air.

Laminar Airflow. Air in a confined area that moves with uniform velocity along parallel lines. The concept was developed by Willis Whitfield of the Sandia Corporation in 1961.

Laminar Airflow Workbenches (LAFWs). The most commonly used PEC that provide ISO Class 5 air or better through either horizontal or vertical unidirectional HEPA-filtered airflows.

Line of Demarcation (LOD). A visible line on the floor that separates the room into areas for different purposes. For example, in the ante-area, the line separates the cleaner area from the clean area of the room.

Malt Extract Agar (MEA). Growth medium that supports fungal growth.

Master Formulation Record. The "recipe" for preparing a CSP that details how the CSP is to be prepared.

Media Fill/Media Transfer. A process for checking aseptic technique or validating a compounding process in which all normal compounding manipulations are performed using a special media instead of the drug. The media will support the growth of many organisms, including some fungi and mold.

Membrane Filtration. A type of sterility testing where the CSP is filtered through a 0.45-micron membrane; the membrane is then aseptically cut in 2 and each half is added to a different type of media.

Multiple-Dose Container. A container of sterile medication for parenteral administration that is designed to contain more than 1 dose of the medication. It is usually required to meet the antimicrobial effectiveness testing criteria.

Negative Pressure. When the air pressure outside a room or vessel is higher than the air pressure inside the room or vessel.

NIOSH. National Institute of Occupational Safety and Health. NIOSH maintains a list of HDs used in the health care setting, which is broken out into different tables based on the risk of the HD. The NIOSH list also provides the criteria used to identify HDs, as drugs may enter the market after the publication of the list, or the organization may handle an investigational drug.

Non-Critical Site. An area that does not provide a pathway between the CSP and the environment.

Open System. A system of holding and transferring solutions that allows air to pass freely in and out, such as using a syringe to extract solution from a broken ampule.

Parenteral Preparations/Solutions. Substances that are introduced to the body by intravenous, subcutaneous, intramuscular, or intramedullary injection.

Pharmacy Bulk Package. A conventionally manufactured sterile product for parenteral use that contains many single doses intended for use in a pharmacy admixture program. It may either be used to prepare admixtures for infusion or, through a sterile transfer device, for filling sterile containers.

Photometer. An instrument used in measuring the intensity of light.

Plenum. The space between the pre-filter and the HEPA filter where air is pressurized and distributed over the HEPA filter.

Positive Pressure. When the air pressure outside a room or vessel is lower than the air pressure inside the room or vessel.

Pre-Filter. A filter that protects the HEPA filter from premature clogging by intercepting larger particles as they enter the laminar airflow.

Primary Engineering Control (PEC). Devices that provide ISO 5 Class air cleanliness for sterile compounding and must: provide unidirectional airflow, supply HEPA-filtered air at a velocity capable of sweeping particles away from critical sites and be placed in a way to accommodate cleaning around and under the device.

Pressure Differential. Pressure between adjacent doorways and rooms that is necessary to ensure consistent airflow from an area of higher air quality to an area of equal or lower air quality.

Protective Over-Wrap. A protective cover, usually plastic, that is sealed over an IV bag.

Quality. The characteristics of a product or service that bear on its ability to meet stated or implied needs, or a product or service free of deficiencies.

Quality Assurance (USP definition). A system of procedures, activities, and oversight that ensures that the compounding process consistently meets quality standards.

Quality Control (USP definition). The sampling, testing, and documentation of results that, taken together, ensure that specifications have been met before release of the CSP.

Quality Management. Oversight of an organization to achieve the desired outcomes.

Quality Management System. The system implements to achieve the desired outcomes.

Repackaging. Transfer of a sterile product or preparation from its original container into another.

Restricted Access Barrier Systems (RABS). Enclosed workspaces that provide vertical airflow, HEPA-filtered ISO Class 5 unidirectional air flow with designed openings that are validated to prevent further transfer of air contamination. These devices have 2 chambers—a main and a transfer chamber—which are used to move materials in and out of the device without introducing contamination.

Sabouraud Dextrose Agar (SDA). Growth medium that supports fungal growth.

Sanitizer. An agent for reducing, on inanimate surfaces, the number of forms of microbial life including fungi, viruses, and bacteria.

Secondary Engineering Control (SEC). Term used for the clean room suite or segregated compounding area (SCA) that are different in design and function and affect the BUD that can be assigned to a CSP.

Segregated Compounding Area (SCA). Designated spaces or rooms in which a PEC may be placed for the preparation of non-hazardous medications.

Single-Dose Container. A container of sterile medication for parenteral administration that is designed for use with a single patient as a single injection/ infusion. It usually does not contain a preservative.

Sporicidal Cleaning Agent. A product that destroys bacterial and fungal spores.

Sterilization. The process that destroys or eliminates all forms of microbial life.

Triple Clean. Cleaning of a target surface 3 times.

Total Particle Count Testing. Used to determine the ISO Class air cleanliness of an area under dynamic conditions and performed using a calibrated particle counter and measures particles 0.5 microns and larger in size.

Trypticase Soy Agar (TSA). General growth medium for both viable and surface samples that supports the growth of bacteria, yeast, and mold.

Validation. Establishing documented evidence that provides a high degree of assurance that a specific process will consistently produce a preparation meeting its predetermined specifications and quality attributes.

Vertical Laminar Airflow Workbench (VLAFW). Like the HLAFW but the air is blown vertically, from the top of the workbench onto the work surface, rather than across.

Visual Smoke Study. Required in a clean room suite if the return exhausts are not located low on a wall and is performed under dynamic conditions to ensure an absence of stagnant airflow in which particles can accumulate.

ABOUT THE AUTHOR

Abby Roth BS, CMQ/OE, microbiologist, and founder of Pure Microbiology, has over 17 years of experience in supporting the testing and consulting needs of the pharmaceutical, medical device, and compounding industries. Her background in pharmaceutical microbiology includes extensive knowledge of environmental monitoring and product testing. Roth also has experience in consulting on microbiological contamination sources and remediation and has been a faculty member on NHIA's Sterile Compounding Workshops. She served on the USP Expert Panel on Sterile Compounding and is an active member of the Controlled Environment Testing Association (CETA). Roth earned a bachelor of science in Biology with a minor in Chemistry from York College of Pennsylvania.

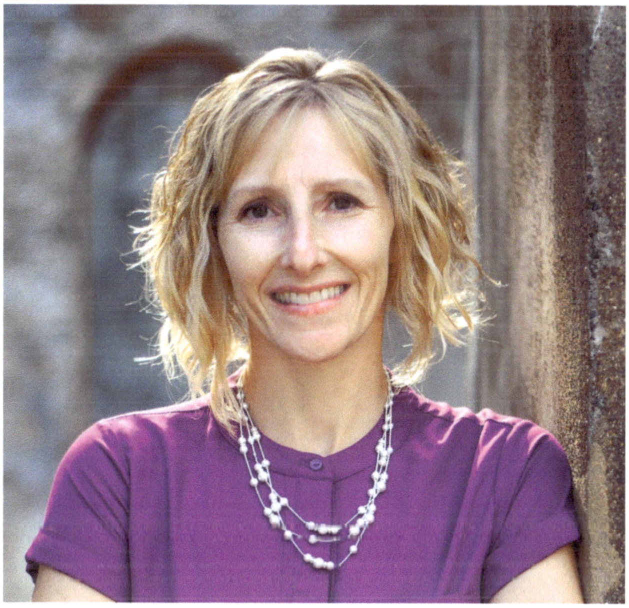

www.ingramcontent.com/pod-product-compliance
Lightning Source LLC
Chambersburg PA
CBHW041828180926
51615CB00005BA/10
* 9 7 8 0 9 8 8 3 0 9 0 5 0 *